Helminthiasis

Edited by Omolade Olayinka Okwa

Published in London, United Kingdom

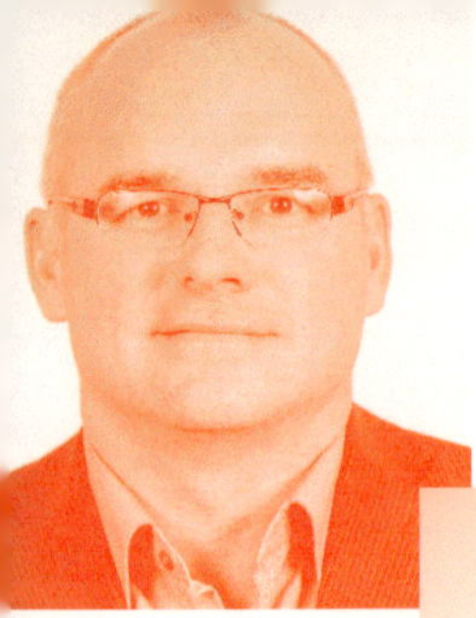
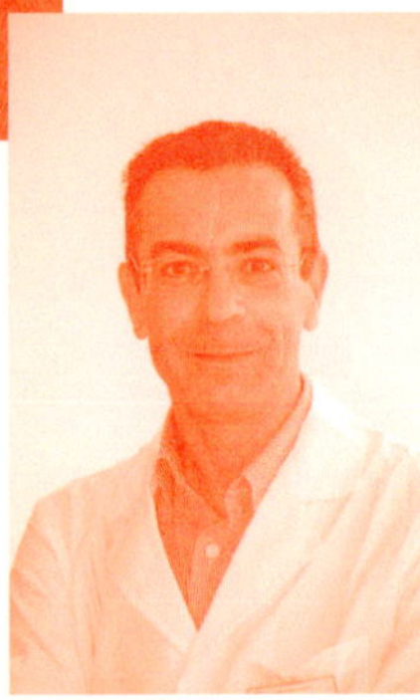
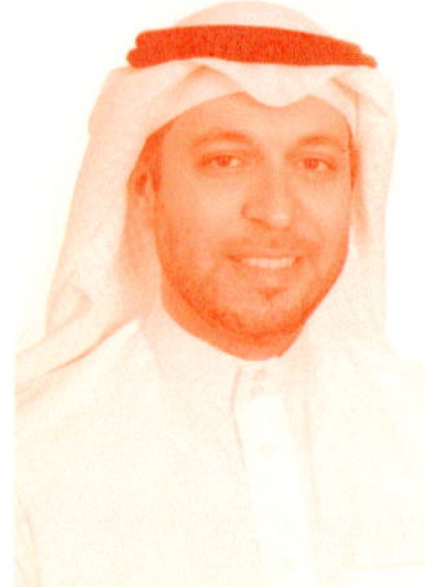
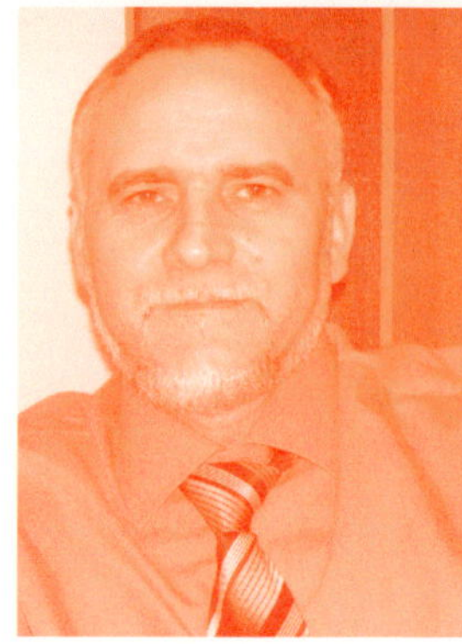
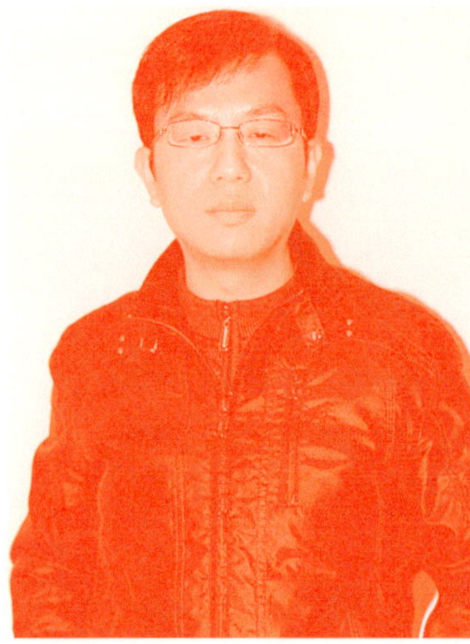
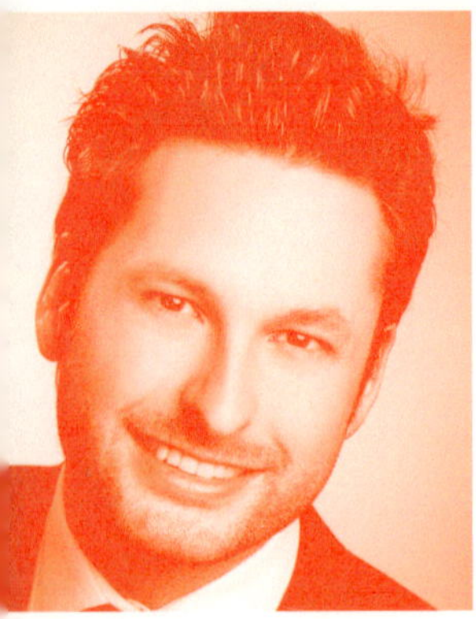
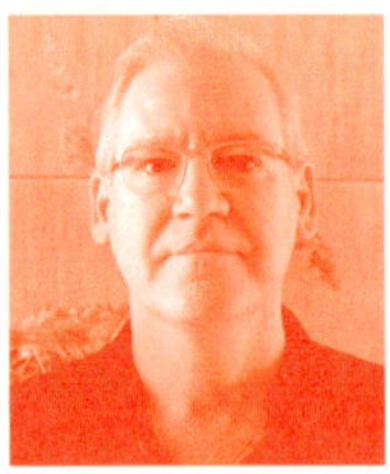

IntechOpen

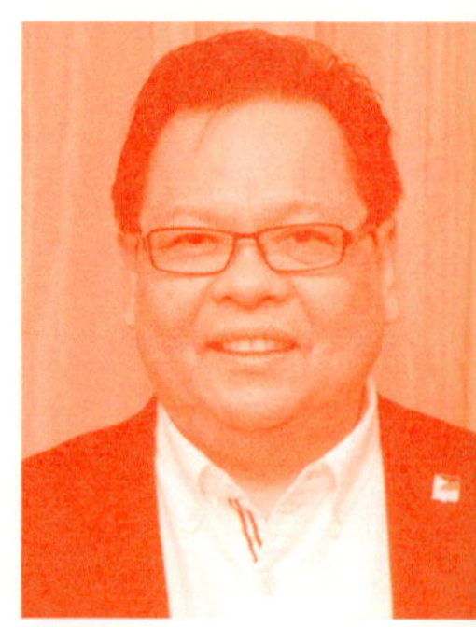
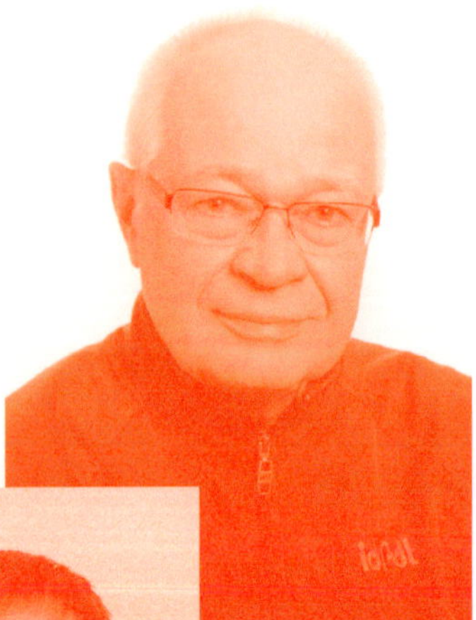
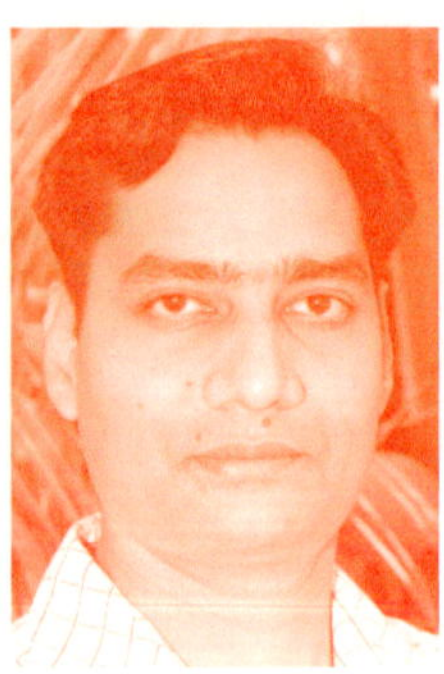
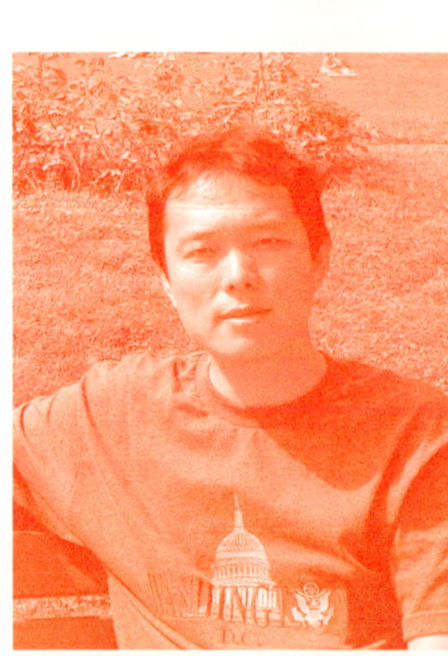
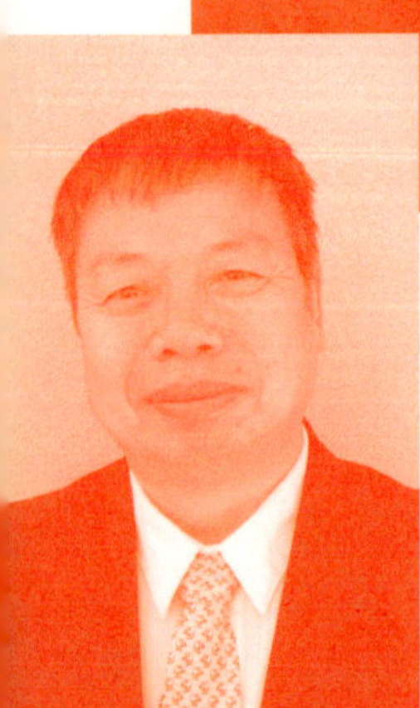
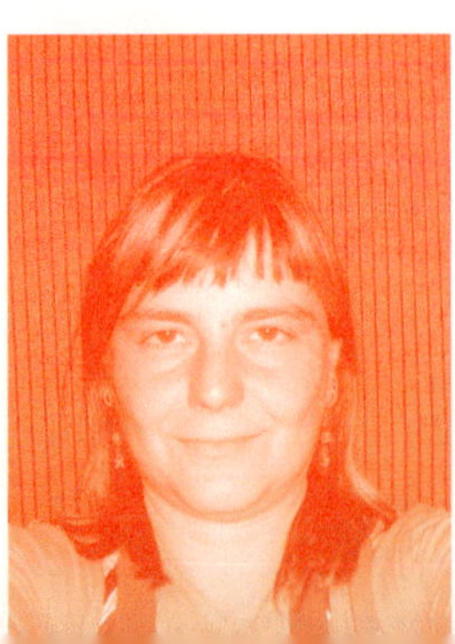

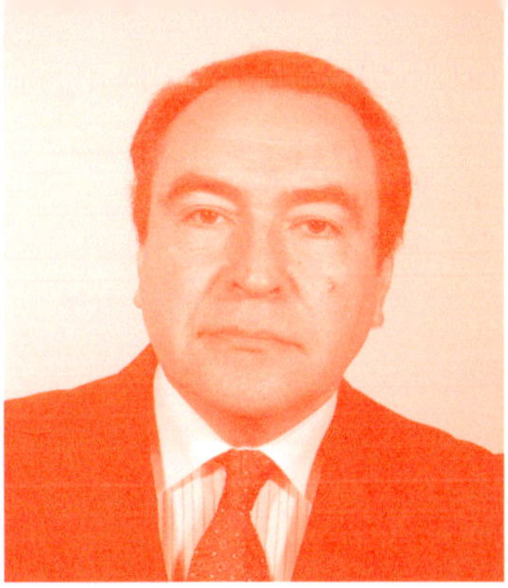
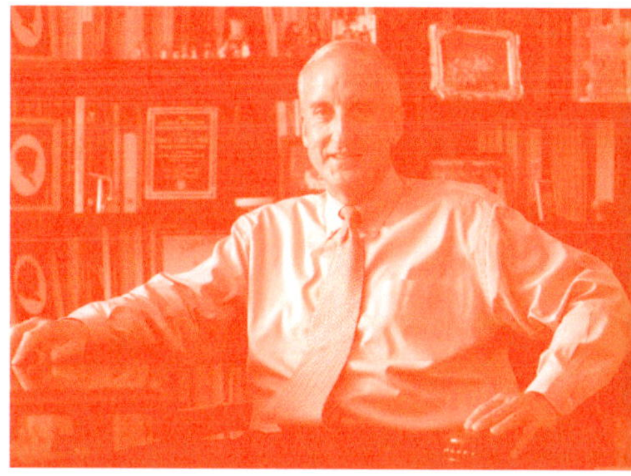
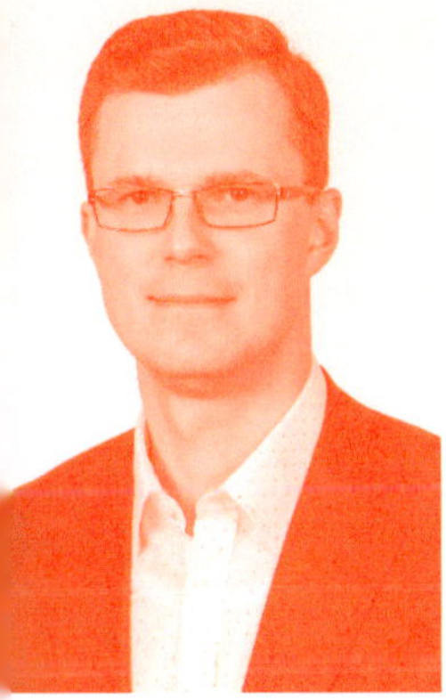
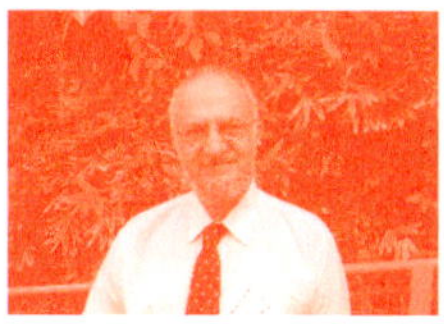
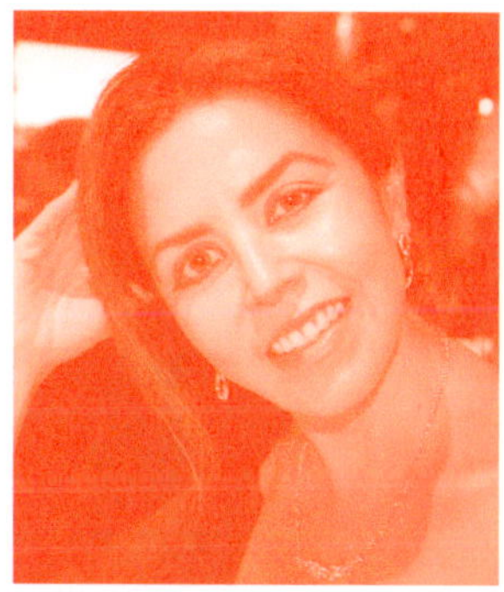

Supporting open minds since 2005

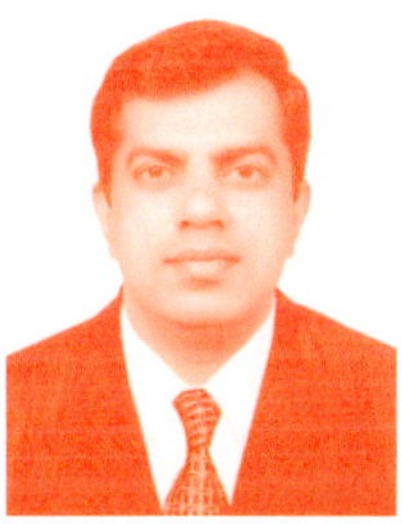
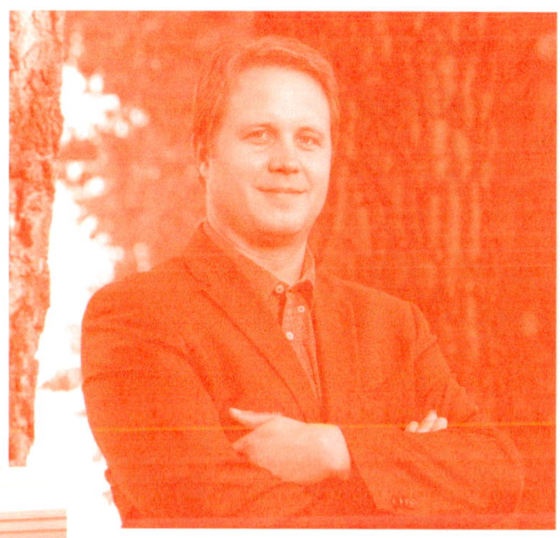
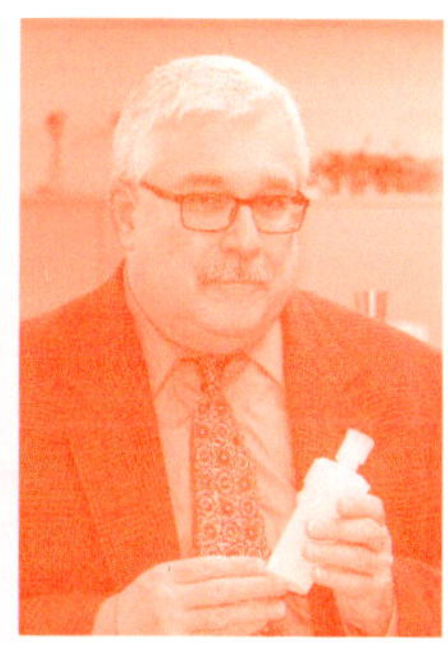
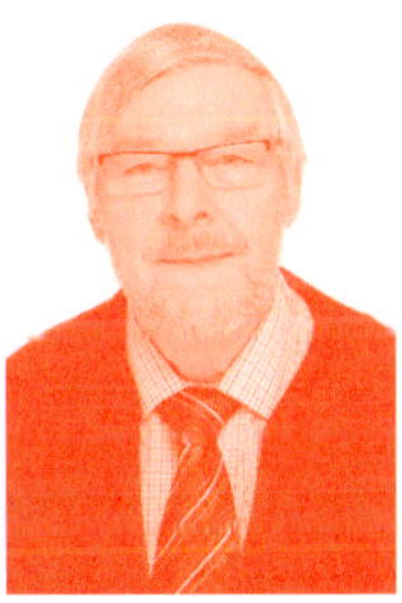
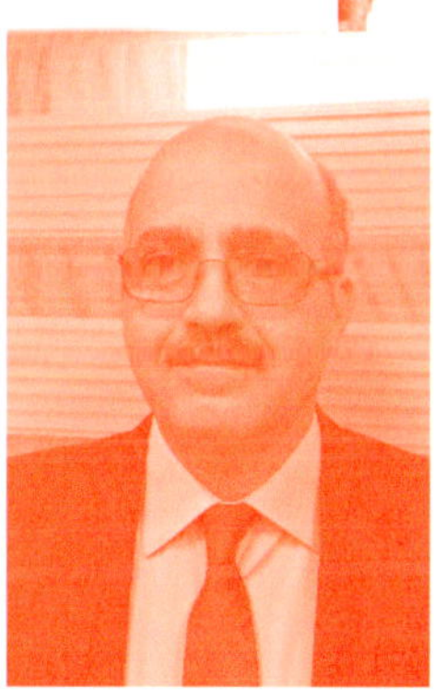
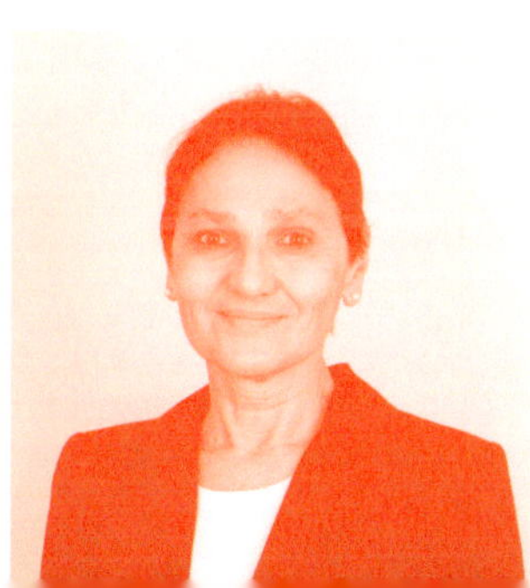
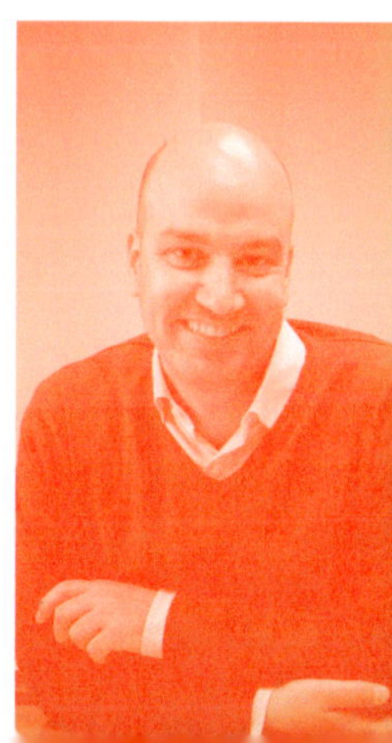

Helminthiasis
http://dx.doi.org/10.5772/intechopen.80144
Edited by Omolade Olayinka Okwa

Contributors
Ingrid Papajová, Jindřich Šoltys, Sharba Kausar, Richard R. Roach, Thekisoe Oriel, Morutse Mphahlele, Nthatisi Molefe, Ana Tsotetsi-Khambule, Neeraj Upmanyu, Asher John Mohan, Silviya Sarah Lal, Omolade Olayinka Okwa

First published in London, United Kingdom, 2020 by IntechOpen
IntechOpen is the global imprint of INTECHOPEN LIMITED, registered in England and Wales, registration number: 11086078, 7th floor, 10 Lower Thames Street, London, EC3R 6AF, United Kingdom
Printed in Croatia

British Library Cataloguing-in-Publication Data
A catalogue record for this book is available from the British Library

Additional hard and PDF copies can be obtained from orders@intechopen.com

Helminthiasis
Edited by Omolade Olayinka Okwa
p. cm.
Print ISBN 978-1-78985-335-3
Online ISBN 978-1-78985-336-0
eBook (PDF) ISBN 978-1-83880-663-7

For EU product safety concerns:
IN TECH d.o.o., Prolaz Marije Krucifikse Kozulić 3, 51000 Rijeka, Croatia, info@intechopen.com or visit our website at intechopen.com.

Meet the editor

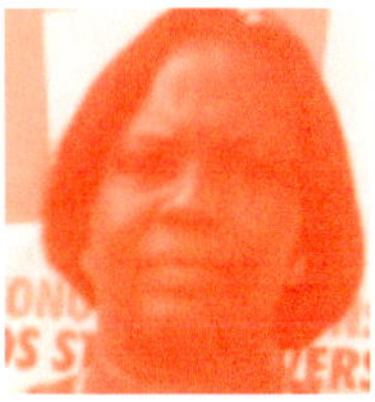

Omolade Olayinka Okwa is presently a Professor of Parasitology at Lagos State University, Nigeria. She has a PhD in Parasitology (1997), an MSc in Cellular Parasitology (1992), and a BSc (Hons) Zoology (1990) all from the University of Ibadan, Nigeria. She teaches parasitology at the undergraduate and postgraduate levels. She was a recipient of a Commonwealth fellowship supported by British Council tenable at the Centre for Entomology and Parasitology (CAEP), Keele University, United Kingdom between 2004 and 2005. She was awarded an Honorary Visiting Research Fellow at the same university from 2005 to 2007. She has been an external examiner to the Department of Veterinary Microbiology and Parasitology, University of Ibadan, MSc programme between 2010 and 2012. She is a member of the Nigerian Society of Experimental Biology (NISEB), Parasitology and Public Health Society of Nigeria (PPSN), Science Association of Nigeria (SAN), Zoological Society of Nigeria (ZSN), and is Vice Chairperson of the Organisation of Women in Science (OWSG), LASU chapter. She served as Head of Department of Zoology and Environmental Biology, Lagos State University from 2007 to 2010 and 2014 to 2016. She is a reviewer for several local and international journals such as Unilag Journal of Science, Libyan Journal of Medicine, Journal of Medicine and Medical Sciences, and Annual Research and Review in Science.
She has authored 45 scientific research publications in local and international journals, 8 scientific reviews, 4 books, and 3 book chapters, which includes the books "Malaria Parasites" and "Malaria" which are IntechOpen access publications.

Contents

Preface

Diseases caused by parasitic helminths (helminthiasis) are infectious and they pose serious health problems, especially in underdeveloped and developing countries of the world. This is a reflection of poor socio-economic conditions, which impacts on the social life of victims and the economic development of affected regions. Helminthiasis is caused by helminths such as flukes, tapeworms, filarial worms, pinworms, thread worms, and soil-transmitted nematodes. Infectious helminths live in a large variety of habitats in humans and other vertebrate hosts.

Helminths are far more widespread than we think. Gastrointestinal helminths (GIHs) are the largest group of helminths that affect man, which results in major threats particularly in underdeveloped and developing countries where they are incorrectly classified as 'Neglected tropical diseases' (NTDS). However, it is a myth to assume that helminths do not exist in temperate countries. GIHs are usually soil-transmitted helminths (STHs) or geohelminths, affecting one third of the world population directly through fecal-oral routes.

The World Health Organization (WHO) reported that about 2.9 million people are infected with gastrointestinal nematodes yearly. A more recent estimate indicates 3.5 billion cases worldwide. About 125,000 deaths are estimated to occur yearly mainly due to STHs. The prevalence of STHs has remained unchanged in over 50 years with 39 million disability adjusted life years (DALYS) lost to these parasites.

> Globally, filariasis, which is vector-transmitted, is the second leading cause of a permanent and long-term disabling and disfiguring disease in the world causing chronic suffering but rarely mortality. According to WHO, in 2002, the DALYS from filariasis was 6 million. In 2013, 1.3 billion people in 72 countries were within areas of endemic filariasis and are continually threatened while an estimated 120 million are already infected.
>
> Control efforts in some communities in underdeveloped and developing countries are impaired by poor sanitation, poverty, and ignorance leading to a high rate of infections and eventually to grave public health challenges. This is why such areas suffer serious consequences due to helminthiasis compared to developed areas. Large scale control programs are essential in less developed countries.

This book provides insights into antihelminthic resistance in livestock, STHs with a focus on pregnant women and children, and what should be done to prevent and control helminth infections for which proper and adequate diagnosis is crucial.

Large scale targeted chemotherapy that focuses on the distribution of safe and effective drugs is an important component of helminthiasis control. This must be complemented with sustainable environmental sanitation and health education to produce a significant reduction in the transmission of helminth infections, especially in the tropics. Hand washing is a major way to prevent parasitic helminth contamination and transmission. This book has helped to close the information gap on helminthiasis, which has otherwise been overlooked as a serious cause of morbidity and mortality of man and animals.

Omolade Olayinka Okwa (Ph.d, CWF)
Associate Professor,
Department of Zoology and Environmental Biology,
Faculty of Science,
Lagos State University,
Nigeria

Section 1

Introductory Chapter

Chapter 1

Introductory Chapter: Helminthes Diversity - Focus on Nematodes

Omolade Olayinka Okwa

1. Introduction

Parasitic helminthes are worms of great medical and veterinary importance. They include the Nematodes (Roundworms) and the Platyhelminthes (Flatworms) which consist of the Trematodes (Flukes) and Cestodes (Tapeworms). These invertebrates are agents of debilitating, deforming and fatal diseases of humans and their agricultural animals and so responsible for great morbidity and mortality. Domestic and wild animals affected by a barrage of helminthes infections may also transmit these infections to humans by zoonoses [1, 2].

Helminthes infections may be vectored, food or water borne. Infections due to parasitic helminthes are no doubt widespread in tropical as well as temperate regions with both regions having their own share of peculiar and distinctive infections. In fact, in Tropical Africa, helminthiasis is regarded as part of the "Neglected tropical diseases" [1].

The platyhelminthes (flatworms) are acoelomates that possess the beginning of some advanced features of the animal kingdom such as cephalization, bilateral symmetry and triploblastic body organization. The trematodes or flukes are endoparasitic platyhelminthes with complex life cycles. The Digeneans are a peculiar group of trematodes in having mollusca (snails) as their intermediate hosts in a life cycle involving one or two hosts; for example: *Schistosoma haematobium* and *Schistosoma mansoni* (blood flukes of man), *Fasciola hepatica* and *Fasciola gigantica* (sheep and cattle liver flukes) and *Paragonimus westermani* (human lung fluke).

Cestodes differ in a number of ways from other flatworms. Their bodies are elongated, ribbon-like and flattened, made up of many segments called proglottids. Most cestodes require at least two hosts of which vertebrates are usually the intermediate host [2]. All these features are adaptations to their exclusively parasitic mode of existence; for example, *Taenia solium* and *Taenia saginata* (pork and beef tapeworms of man), *Echinococcus granulosus* and *Echinococcus multilocularis* (dog tapeworms) and *Diphyllobothrium latum* (broad fish tapeworm of man).

2. Nematodes (the roundworms)

2.1 The ubiquity of nematodes

Nematodes are cosmopolitan and ubiquitous. They are one of the most numerous metazoans in the animal kingdom with broad ranges of environment having successfully adapted to every ecosystem both aquatic and terrestrial. They are a large group of bilaterally symmetrical, elongated, pseudocoelomate helminthes in the animal kingdom. They are elongated, non-metamerically segmented, and cylindrical or round so referred to as the round worms. *Nema* from the word Nematode means thread because they are threadlike, vermiform and slender worms [1]. They are the largest and the most successful pseudocoelomate phylum and very remarkable organisms. It has been estimated that the total number of nematode species might be approximately 1,000,000 in about 20 orders within two classes [3]. It is believed that 90% of animals on the ocean floor and 80% of animals on earth may be nematodes. It is believed that a handful of soil contains hundreds of nematodes and that soil habitats may contain undescribed free-living nematodes [4].

2.2 Parasitic nematodes

Most nematodes are free-living but over 16,000 are parasitic and cause infections leading to great morbidity and mortality to humans, animals and plants [2].

For example, some nematodes are directly transmitted through the soil which harbors their eggs and larvae stages and hence called the soil transmitted helminthes. Such nematodes are *Ascaris lumbricoides* (common roundworm of man), *Trichuris trichiura* (whipworm), *Necator americanus* and *Ancylostoma duodenalis* (hookworms of man) and *Strongyloides stercoralis* (thread worm of man) [5, 6].

Some nematodes are indirectly transmitted as they require vectors usually arthropods for them to be transmitted from one host to another as in the filarial worms such as *Loa loa* (African eye worm), *Onchocerca volvulus, Wuchereria bancrofti* and *Brugia* species.

Some nematodes are parasitic in animals, for example, *Ascaris suum* (pig), *Ascaridia galli* (chicken), *Toxocara canis, Trichuris vulpis* and *Strongyloides canis* (dogs), *Ancylostoma tubaeforme* and *A. brazilense* (cat hookworms) [7].

2.3 Types of parasitic nematodes

Nematode parasites can reside in every tissue in their vertebrate host. Therefore, they can be categorized according to their residence in their host [8, 9]:

- **Intestinal nematodes**: they are usually large nematodes transmitted directly to the host and dwelling in the gastrointestinal tract, e.g., *Ascaris lumbricoides, Trichuris trichiura, Hookworms, Strongyloides stercoralis,* and *Enterobius vermicularis.* Polyparasitism of enteric nematodes has been documented [1].

- **Soil-transmitted nematodes** (geohelminths): these are nematodes whose eggs embryonate in the soil and larvae stages also undergo ecdysis in the soil and are transmitted directly to the host, e.g., *Ascaris lumbricoides, Trichuris trichiura*, *Necator americanus* and *Ancylostoma duodenale* (hookworms).

- **Filarial nematodes:** these are thread like nematodes that have a pre-larval stage call microfilaria and are transmitted indirectly via an insect vector to the host which are usually mammals, e.g., *Onchocerca volvulus*, *Loa loa, Wuchereria bancrofti, Brugia malayi, Brugia timori* and *Dipetalonema streptocerca*.

- **Tissue dwelling nematodes:** these are nematodes living in the tissues of the host such as in the lymphatics, e.g., *Wuchereria bancrofti, Brugia malayi* and *Dracunculus medinensis* (serous tissue).

- **Subcutaneous nematodes**: these consist of nematode dwelling in the subcutaneous tissue of their host, e.g., *Onchocerca volvulus, Loa loa, Mansonella perstans*.

3. General transmission and reproduction patterns of nematodes

Nematodes have diverse modes of transmission strategies and great variation in life cycles which are complex. Nematodes are gonochoristic with distinct separate sexes. They have larger females than males, which possess copulatory spicules for internal fertilization. They have tubular gonads and amoeboid sperm cells. Only very few nematodes are monoecious [5, 6].

Some nematodes are parthenogenetic such as threadworms. Most are oviparous such as *Ascaris lumbricoides* (common roundworm), *Trichuris trichiura* (whipworm) and *Enterobius vermicularis* (pinworm). Ovoviviparous nematodes include threadworms and hookworms because they lay eggs with larvae. Viviparous nematodes are *Trichinella spiralis*, filarial worms and *Dracunculus medinensis* (Guinea worm) because they give rise directly to larvae [5–7].

Nematodes are long lived worms with highly resistant eggs and great fecundity (large egg outputs) which is adaptive to juvenile survival. Their eggs exhibit remarkable uniformity in size ranging from 50 to 90 μm long. However, the egg shells are highly variable but basically have three to five layers and are highly resistant to environmental conditions. Nematodes have life cycles with larval stages that resemble the adults. The larval stages have four molts and one adult basically (egg-L_1-L_2-L_3-adult) [1, 2].

3.1 Adaptations of parasitic nematodes

These are features that make their parasitic existence a success and they include the:

- **Body wall and pseudocoel**: this protects the worm in the host environment which is the small intestine. The epidermis is a syncytium consisting of a single layer of cells, covered by a thick collagenous cuticle. The complex and metabolically active cuticle often have two or three distinct layers. Underneath the epidermis, lies a layer of longitudinal muscle cells. The pseudocoel acts as hydrostatic skeleton [6, 7].

- **Digestive system:** the digestive systems are highly efficient for parasitic mode of life. The oral cavity opens into a muscular sucking pharynx, also lined with cuticle. They have complete digestive system, referring to the alimentary canal which extends from the anterior mouth to the anus located near the tail. The mouth has lips in some cases.

- **Reproductive system**: this is adaptive to the survival of the parasites. Sexes in nematodes are separate and they have complex life cycles. They have prodigious fecundity and eggs are often highly resistant to desiccation. The eggs are protected by an outer shell, secreted by the uterus. The larval stages resemble the adults and undergo 4 molts (first to third stage larvae). The third stage larva is usually infective and can respond to a wide range of stimuli before it molts to adult in the host [1, 2].

4. Conclusion

Helminthiasis, no doubt consists of a group of diseases of important public health and socio-economic significance so it is a paradox to be described as "Neglected tropical diseases." The cosmopolitan, ubiquitous and adaptive nature of nematodes and other helminthes are far more than we often think. This gives reasons to suggest that helminthiasis should not be underestimated as a serious cause of morbidity and mortality.

Author details

Omolade Olayinka Okwa
Department of Zoology, Lagos State University, Lagos, Nigeria

*Address all correspondence to: okwaomolade@hotmail.com

References

[1] Ukoli FMA. Introduction to Parasitology in Tropical Africa. Ibadan, Nigeria: Text Flow Publishers; 1990. p. 462. ISBN: 978-2783-005

[2] Okwa OO. The Biology of the Tropical Parasites. Germany: Lambert Academic Publishers; 2016. p. 145. ISBN: 978-3-330-00888-5

[3] Otubanjo OA. Parasites of Man and Animals. Lagos, Nigeria: Concept Publications; 2013. p. 648. ISBN: 978-978-51446-04; 419-558

[4] Anderson RC. Nematode Parasites of Vertebrates: Their Development and Transmission. 2nd ed. Oxford, UK: CABI Publishing; 2000. p. 650. ISBN: 085198799-0

[5] Hugot P, Banjard P, Morano S. Biodiversity in helminthes as a field of study: An overview. Nematology. 2001;**3**:199-208

[6] Smyth JD. Introduction to Animal Parasitology. 3rd ed. Cambridge, UK: Cambridge University Press; 1994. p. 549. ISBN: 0521-428114

[7] World Health Organization. Global Burden of Diseases. Geneva: WHO Technical Report; 2008. p. 160. ISBN: 978-924-1563710

[8] Da Silva NR, Booker S, Hotex PJ, Montressor A, Eagles D, Savioli L. Soil transmitted helminthes. Updating the global picture. Trends in Parasitology. 2003;**19**:547-551

[9] Larry RS, Janovy JJ. Foundations of Parasitology. 8th ed. New York, United States: McGraw Hill; 2009. pp. 120-150

Section 2

Soil Transmitted Helminthes

Chapter 2

Pregnancy, Children and Inter-Relating Factors Affected by Geohelminthiasis

Asher John Mohan, Neeraj Upmanyu and Silviya Sarah Lal

Abstract

A life-threatening parasitic infection arising in evolving countries, principally prevalent in children below 5 years and pregnant women, has led to the growing interest for understanding the condition acknowledged as geohelminthiasis. Decreased cell-mediated immunity (a necessity in fetal retention) leading to a compromised immunological response is what makes pregnant women more prone to the infection thereby increasing the risk of maternal anemia, preterm deliveries and stillbirths based on reports. An outcome of geohelminthiasis on children is its deteriorative effect on cognition. This chapter highlights the relationship between the helminthic infection with respect to pregnant women and children additionally focusing on other associated factors such as poverty, hygiene, etc. that further contribute to the decline in quality of life in developing countries.

Keywords: geohelminthiasis, cell-mediated immunity, cognition, pregnancy, parasitic infection

1. Introduction

The general term used to describe a worm is referred to as a "helminth." These invertebrates fall under two categories, namely flatworms or Platyhelminthes (flukes and tapeworms) and roundworms or Nematoda [1, 2]. They either survive in aquatic and terrestrial environments as parasites or free of a host. Out of the various types, intestinal nematodes or soil-transmitted helminths (STH) also known as "Geohelminths" are the most common worldwide. The World Health Organization (WHO) claims that 1.5 billion people worldwide, constituting to 24% of the world's population, are infected by STH; with wide distributions in the Sub-Saharan Africa, America, China and East Asia in tropical and subtropical regions [3].

The major infection of STH originates from the attack of *Ascaris lumbricoides* (commonly called the large intestinal roundworm or the common roundworm) and *Trichuris trichiura* (whipworm) [4, 5]. Hookworm (Ancylostomatidae) affliction is also another most common chronic infection found in humans that contribute to STH [6].

Children are the frequent victims to an STH attack as many of them are school aged, living in areas of extensive disease transmission; requiring treatment interventions and preventive measures [7]. Secondary victims of this infection are pregnant women reported every year, among which 44 million are estimated to be affected globally [8]. Improvements in potable water services, drainage, sanitary food control, living quarters, individual and community anti-vector action are a few conceptualizations that can be implemented for the eradication of this infectious outbreak [9].

The central focus of this chapter is to gain insight into as to how aspects of childhood and pregnancy are concomitant to geohelminthiasis, along with various other inter-relating factors such as poverty, hygiene, etc.; that cause a drop in the quality of life in developing countries.

2. Immune responses to STH

Preclinical data from animals suggest that th2 (T-helper) cells are triggered by cytokine release along with immunoglobulin E (IgE) of the host immune system aiding in the elimination of helminthic burdens [10, 11]. However, the innate and adaptive immunity are often markedly found to remain suppressed. This indicates that immune responses triggered due to a helminthic infection could result in host protection responses against microbial pathogens to be antagonized [12, 13]. Recent findings of the involvement of macrophages referred to as alternatively activated macrophages can also be a contributing factor leading to an inflammatory response when in contact with a helminth [14].

3. Children and geohelminthiasis

School children of countries affected by this epidemic, were found to exhibit the greatest incidence and severity of the outbreak. No ill effects (with respect to morbidity) were thought to be experienced by children with light infections. However, recent evidences oppose this traditional notion with reports of slight or minimal intensity outbreaks having significant decrement in the development and growth of children [15]. Information regarding as to how various factors affect geohelminthiasis in children is discussed below.

3.1 Nutrition

Nutrition plays a key role as a target for the alleviation of helminthic infections. Several surroundings of the developing world are impacted by malnutrition and helminthic infection, both as their main or supplementary factors governing mortality [16]. Impaired digestion, malabsorption, diminution in food consumption and poor growth rates are often noted in children who endure this helminthic incursion [17]. Recent studies also depict the fact that malnutrition is in direct proportion to the intensity of the pathogen Ascaris [18]. Other factors governing infection scale include the extent of nutritional deficiency and concurrent prominence of single or multiple infections and single or multiple nutritional deficiencies [19]. Increased loss of endogenic protein paired with the distress of energy and mineral metabolism are the mechanisms by which an intestinal nematode reduces feed intake by the host. Better nutrition can improve the rate of adult worm rejection via an approach of diet consumption rich in metabolizable proteins [20].

The improvement of the nutritional status of school children would be an essential remedy for disease alleviation [21, 22].

3.2 Environment

The environmental variables attributing to the risk of this parasitic outbreak cannot be avoided as a correlation between this aspect and disease condition is of high prevalence.

Recent studies of various schools reporting the presence of certain other influential environmental factors governing the infection such an inadequate water supply, requirement of regular water/sanitation maintenance regimes and overcrowding in classrooms can be taken into consideration for disease management [23].

3.3 Anti-helminthic treatment in children

Since the primary mode of therapy includes the use of anti-helminthics, development of resistance due to their administration is a crucial factor governing geohelminthiasis. The known variables that add value to an anti-helminthic resistance are medication frequency, refuge or the percentage in the parasite population not exposed to drugs and the possibility of underdosing [24].

Another causative factor in children leading to intestinal obstruction observed was prior anti-helminthic treatment [25]. Although specific IgE antibodies are believed to participate in the protection against helminthic infection, the polyclonal stimulation of IgE caused by helminthic parasites could be the sole reason for re-infection [26]. In a follow-up investigation concerning growth retarded children where anti-helminthic therapy was discontinued after successful alleviation; the extent of re-infection was found to dramatically increase which could pose difficulty in the quality of life of the concerned [27].

3.4 Cognition

The negative influence of STH infections on cognitive processes, notably in school children; has been deduced by researchers since 1900. Prolonged anemia and toxemia were factors accountable for the substantial increase in the degree of cognitive delay with respect to the level of infection. However, clarification remains to be produced regarding the mechanism by which worms impact cognition. Certain postulates comprise of malnutrition and fatigue in children troubled from the infection as consequences of diminished cognition. Reports of medication reversing this adverse effect are also at large and very much essential for effective control of the disease [28–30].

4. Pregnancy and geohelminthiasis

Helminthic infections are suggested to be extremely damaging, with detrimental effects on maternal anemia and birth outcomes in cases of pregnancy, with a total global impact on pregnancies estimated to be 44 million [31, 32].

4.1 Probable mechanism of susceptibility to STH in pregnancy

A characteristic feature of pregnancy is the successful retention of the fetus due to hormonal, dietary and immunological changes occurring during the period [33]. This is a unique illustration of how the body adjusts to a destructive immune response during pregnancy [34]. Therefore, studies have clearly defined the characteristic of pregnancy as immune modulation and not its suppression. In other words, an alteration to the immune system contributes to differential responses not merely on the basis of microorganisms but on the basis of stage of pregnancy [35].

Although the periparturic immunosuppression involvement remains unclear, one of the proposed mechanism depicts the avoidance of particular processes of host immune defense by the parasitic helminth [36, 37]. The resemblance between the immune reactions to helminths and pregnant females may be a sign that tolerance may be invoked by analogous mechanisms (i.e., type 2 responses). Another suggestion has been that helminths may have undergone self-adaptation in order to combat immune responses from the mother by utilizing the similarity in mechanisms as used by a human fetus [38]. These could have been some among the many reasons a pregnant mother's susceptibility to helminthic attack is widespread.

The WHO reports that far more than half of the pregnant females in emerging economies have concerns pertaining to iron deficiency anemia, which could be a result of an elevated metabolic requisite for iron during childbirth coupled with poor nutrition. This iron STH related deficiency has been concomitant to augmented mortality rate, premature birth and low birth weights during the period of pregnancy [39, 40].

4.2 Co-infection

Considering pregnancy, the susceptibility to co-infections cannot be ignored due to immunological modulations associated with the stage. Data indicating the exhibition of higher prevalence of *Trichuris trichiura*, followed by an *Ascaris lumbricoides* infection were found in cases of pregnancy; where attacks of a single infection was found to be at a higher percent than that of co-infections [41]. Considering co-infections associated with pregnancy related STH, it was found that the malarial parasite *Plasmodium falciparum* co-existed with hookworms, when compared to roundworms and whipworms [42, 43].

4.3 Geophagy (soil eating)

Another causal component for STH diseases is geophagy that is practiced among some African females. While the exact reason remains a mystery, some beliefs such as curing heartburn and alleviating morning sickness are still at large [44]. Adequate data indicates that geophagy can be associated with enhanced anemic peril and reduced hemoglobin amounts [45]. Geophagy in lactating mothers resulted in reinfection and hence was advised for immediate interventions to tackle disease transmission [46].

4.4 Maternal anemia

The greater the severity of hookworm infestations, the greater was the percentage of blood loss or anemia observed in pregnant women from an endemic area survey [47]. During pregnancy, the hookworm, in particular, was considered to be the source of mild associative anemia while the other STH's were involved in mild deficiencies of iron [48, 49]. A current connection between co-infection and anemia, as reported in the latest studies indicate that the latter is not a sole companion of helminthic attack alone [50].

Since there is an additional relationship between anemia and birth outcomes (increased risk of preterm birth or low birth weight), a helminthic outbreak could also be affiliated to the second during pregnancy [51]. All the above findings indicate that the association of anemia due to STH can be debilitating in case of pregnant women.

4.5 Birth outcomes

The reason for the problem of low birth weight was the exposition to an attack of hookworm resulting in intrauterine growth retardation especially in cases of HIV infected subjects [52]. A lower prevalence of low birth weight was the end result of periodic anti-helminthics and the weekly iron folic acid supplements before pregnancy [53]. Another birth outcome experienced was the premature birth. Similar to the case of maternal anemia, the co-existence of other infections with STH brought about a greater negative birth outcomes.

5. Present beneficial hypotheses

Although helminthic infections are difficult for kids and for pregnant females, the asymptomatic stage in an helminthic infection was found act as a guard keeper against immunological syndromes [54]. An unusual, inflammatory bowel disease (characterized by chronic gastrointestinal inflammation) hygiene hypothesis suggests a lack of exposure to intestinal helminths as an important environmental factor contributing to the development of such illnesses [55, 56].

The possibility of predisposition to Crohn's disease (an inflammatory idiopathic bowel disease, most often involving the ileum, colon and in certain cases; the esophagus) due to lack of exposure to helminthic parasites as per data of a certain study [57, 58]. A similar small cross-sectional study showed the prevalence of STH to have beneficial effects in patients with type 2 diabetes (insulin resistant). However, this may seem to be damaging in areas where helminthic treatment options are a must to curb disease morbidity [59].

6. Other inter-relating factors

All the above discussed variables associated with children and pregnant women are also dependent on conditions of on geographical circumstances, poverty and bad hygiene. The STH assault is restricted to rural regions of tropics, especially in coastal regions; where temperature, humidity and soil type are appropriate for development and growth. Exposure to larval eggs in farming areas where individuals expose their skin to the hot and humid soil is what aids in disease transmission. Sandy soils provide better growth conditions for these worms when compared to clayey soils. An important adverse link between socioeconomic status and incidence or severity of helminthic disease can also attribute towards the spread of STH. It was found that the prevalence of disease was less in cases of higher income groups. Bad sanitation or hygiene due to the lack of income is also an associated factor leading to an attack of STH [60–63].

7. Conclusion

Geohelminthiasis or soil-transmitted helminthiasis is recognized as a life-threatening parasitic outbreak in developing nations, predominantly in kids under 5 years of age and pregnant females and has resulted to increased concern. Reports of nutrition, environment, resistance to treatment and cognition were the associative parameters found in children, whereas in the condition of pregnancy existence of co-infections, geophagy, maternal anemia and birth outcomes were found to be the inter-relating variables to STH. The avoidance of particular processes of host immune defense and self-adaptation to combat immune responses from the mother by utilizing the similarity in mechanisms as used by a human fetus were the proposed mechanisms by which pregnant women are more prone to the attack. All the associative parameters discussed above were found to increase disease burden. Tackling these factors is therefore a must for achieving an improved quality of life.

Although recent or upcoming beneficial hypotheses could play an important role in the eradication of associative diseases, the same benefit could have least highlighting phenomena when poverty is involved. Improvements in hygiene and improved access to anti-helminthic drugs are some of the factors that could establish a better alleviating status for the disease attack. Further researches/studies and proper awareness among groups where the disease is endemic is however still a requisite for both devising and strategizing to fight against the disease.

Acknowledgements

The authors would like to express their gratitude to People's University, Bhanpur, Bhopal, for providing the necessary environment for completion of this chapter.

Conflict of interest

We the authors would like to declare that there is no conflict of interest based on the information produced.

Author details

Asher John Mohan[1*], Neeraj Upmanyu[1] and Silviya Sarah Lal[2]

1 School of Pharmacy and Research, Affiliated to People's University, Bhopal, India

2 Indian Institute of Science Education and Research (IISER), Bhopal, India

*Address all correspondence to: asherjohnmohan@gmail.com

References

[1] Castro GA. Helminths: Structure, classification, growth, and development. In: Baron S, editor. Medical Microbiology. 4th ed. Galveston (TX): University of Texas Medical Branch at Galveston; 1996. Available from: http://www.ncbi.nlm.nih.gov/books/NBK8282/

[2] Wakelin D. Helminths: Pathogenesis and defenses. In: Baron S, editor. Medical Microbiology. 4th ed. Galveston (TX): University of Texas Medical Branch at Galveston; 1996. Available from: http://www.ncbi.nlm.nih.gov/books/NBK8191/

[3] Soil-Transmitted Helminth Infections. 2019. Available from: https://www.who.int/news-room/fact-sheets/detail/soil-transmitted-helminth-infections

[4] Walker M, Hall A, Basáñez M-G. Ascaris lumbricoides: New epidemiological insights and mathematical approaches. In: Holland C, editor. Ascaris: The Neglected Parasite. Amsterdam: Elsevier; 2013. pp. 155-201. Available from: http://www.sciencedirect.com/science/article/pii/B9780123969781000070

[5] Bundy DA, Cooper ES, Brooker S. Nematodes limited to the intestinal tract (*Enterobius vermicularis*, *Trichuris trichiura*, *Capillaria philippinensis* and *Trichostrongylus* spp.). In: Magill AJ, Hill DR, Solomon T, Ryan ET, editors. Hunter's Tropical Medicine and Emerging Infectious Disease. 9th ed. London: W.B. Saunders; 2013. pp. 797-803. Available from: http://www.sciencedirect.com/science/article/pii/B9781416043904001077

[6] Brooker S, Bethony J, Hotez PJ. Human hookworm infection in the 21st century. Advances in Parasitology. 2004;**58**:197-288

[7] Karshima SN. Prevalence and distribution of soil-transmitted helminth infections in Nigerian children: A systematic review and meta-analysis. Infectious Diseases of Poverty. 2018;**7**(1):69

[8] Salam RA, Haider BA, Humayun Q, Bhutta ZA. Effect of administration of antihelminthics for soil-transmitted helminths during pregnancy. Cochrane Database of Systematic Reviews. 2015;**6**:CD005547

[9] Kumate J. Infectious diseases in the 21st century. Archives of Medical Research. 1997;**28**(2):155-161

[10] Maynard CL, Weaver CT. Effector CD4+ T cells in the intestines. In: Mestecky J, Strober W, Russell MW, Kelsall BL, Cheroutre H, Lambrecht BN, editors. Mucosal Immunology. 4th ed. Boston: Academic Press; 2015. pp. 721-732. Available from: http://www.sciencedirect.com/science/article/pii/B9780124158474000343

[11] Carty SA, Riese MJ, Koretzky GA. T-Cell Immunity. In: Hoffman R, Benz EJ, Silberstein LE, Heslop HE, Weitz JI, Anastasi J, et al., editors. Hematology. 9th ed. Elsevier; 2018. p. 221-239. DOI: 10.1016/C2013-0-23355-9. Available from: http://www.sciencedirect.com/science/article/pii/B9780323357623000214

[12] Jackson JA, Friberg IM, Little S, Bradley JE. Review series on helminths, immune modulation and the hygiene hypothesis: Immunity against helminths and immunological phenomena in modern human populations: Coevolutionary legacies? Immunology. 2009;**126**(1):18-27

[13] Salgame P, Yap GS, Gause WC. Effect of helminth-induced immunity on infections with microbial

pathogens. Nature Immunology. 2013;**14**(11):1118-1126

[14] Kreider T, Anthony RM, Urban JF, Gause WC. Alternatively activated macrophages in helminth infections. Current Opinion in Immunology. 2007 Aug;**19**(4):448-453

[15] Zulkifli A, Anuar AK, Atiya A, Yano A. The prevalence of malnutrition and geo-helminth infections among primary schoolchildren in rural kelantan. The Southeast Asian Journal of Tropical Medicine and Public Health. 2000;**31**(2):7

[16] Bundy DAP, Golden MHN. The impact of host nutrition on gastrointestinal helminth populations. Parasitology. 1987;**95**(3):623-635

[17] Crompton DWT, Nesheim MC. Nutritional impact of intestinal helminthiasis during the human life cycle. Annual Review of Nutrition. 2002;**22**(1):35-59

[18] Yamamoto R, Nagai N, Kawabata M, Leon WU, Ninomiya R, Koizumi N. Effect of intestinal helminthiasis on nutritional status of schoolchildren. The Southeast Asian Journal of Tropical Medicine and Public Health. 2000;**31**(4):7

[19] Koski KG, Scott ME. Gastrointestinal nematodes, nutrition and immunity: Breaking the negative spiral. Annual Review of Nutrition. 2001;**21**(1):297-321

[20] Van Houtert MFJ, Sykes AR. Implications of nutrition for the ability of ruminants to withstand gastrointestinal nematode infections. International Journal for Parasitology. 1996;**26**(11):1151-1167

[21] Jemaneh L. Schistosomiasis mansoni and geo-helminthiasis in school children in the Dembia plains, Northwest Ethiopia. The Ethiopian Journal of Health Development. 1998;**12**(3):1-11. Available from: https://www.ejhd.org/index.php/ejhd/article/view/984

[22] Tulu B, Taye S, Zenebe Y, Amsalu E. Intestinal parasitic infections and nutritional status among primary school children in Delo-mena District, South Eastern Ethiopia. Iranian Journal of Parasitology. 2016;**11**(4):549-558

[23] Hughes RG, Sharp DS, Hughes MC, Akauola S, Heinsbroek P, Velayudhan R, et al. Environmental influences on helminthiasis and nutritional status among Pacific schoolchildren. International Journal of Environmental Health Research. 2004;**14**(3):163-177

[24] Vercruysse J, Albonico M, Behnke JM, Kotze AC, Prichard RK, McCarthy JS, et al. Is anthelmintic resistance a concern for the control of human soil-transmitted helminths? International Journal for Parasitology: Drugs and Drug Resistance. 2011;**1**(1):14-27

[25] Anthelmintics as a Risk Factor in Intestinal Obstruction by *Ascaris lumbricoides* in children - Abstract - Europe PMC. 2019. Available from: https://europepmc.org/abstract/med/11757415

[26] Hagel I, Lynch NR, Prisco MCD, Rojas E, Pérez M, Alvarez N. Ascaris reinfection of slum children: Relation with the IgE response. Clinical and Experimental Immunology. 1993;**94**(1):80-83

[27] Hagel I. Helminthic infection and anthropometric indicators in children from a tropical slum: Ascaris reinfection after anthelmintic treatment. Journal of Tropical Pediatrics. 1999;**45**(4):215-220

[28] Nokes C, Grantham-McGregor SM, Sawyer AW, Cooper ES, Bundy DAP. Parasitic helminth infection and cognitive function in school children. Proceedings of the Royal Society of London B. 1992;**247**(1319):77-81

[29] Nokes C, Bundy DAP. Does helminth infection affect mental processing and educational achievement? Parasitology Today. 1994;**10**(1):14-18

[30] Mcgarvey ST, Olveda RM, Acosta LP, Kurtis JD, Bellinger DC, Langdon GC, et al. Helminth infection and cognitive impairment among filipino children. The American Journal of Tropical Medicine and Hygiene. 2005;**72**(5):540-548

[31] Brooker S, Hotez PJ, Bundy DAP. Hookworm-related anaemia among pregnant women: A systematic review. PLoS Neglected Tropical Diseases. 2008;**2**(9). Available from: https://www.ncbi.nlm.nih.gov/pmc/articles/PMC2553481/

[32] Haider BA, Humayun Q, Bhutta ZA. Effect of administration of antihelminthics for soil transmitted helminths during pregnancy. Cochrane Database of Systematic Reviews. 2009;**2**:CD005547

[33] Mpairwe H, Tweyongyere R, Elliott A. Pregnancy and helminth infections. Parasite Immunology. 2014;**36**(8):328-337

[34] Guleria I, Sayegh MH. Maternal acceptance of the fetus: True human tolerance. The Journal of Immunology. 2007;**178**(6):3345-3351

[35] Mor G, Cardenas I. The immune system in pregnancy: A unique complexity. American Journal of Reproductive Immunology. 2010;**63**(6):425-433

[36] Lloyd S. Effect of pregnancy and lactation upon infection. Veterinary Immunology and Immunopathology. 1983;**4**(1-2):153-176

[37] Mulcahy G, O'Neill S, Fanning J, McCarthy E, Sekiya M. Tissue migration by parasitic helminths—An immunoevasive strategy? Trends in Parasitology. 2005;**21**(6):273-277

[38] Blackwell AD. Helminth infection during pregnancy: Insights from evolutionary ecology. International Journal of Women's Health. 2016;**8**:651-661

[39] Hotez PJ, Brooker S, Bethony JM, Bottazzi ME, Loukas A, Xiao S. Hookworm Infection. The New England Journal of Medicine. 2004;**351**(8):799-807

[40] Kalenga MK, Nyembo MK, Nshimba M, Foidart JM. Anemia and associated factors (malaria and intestinal helminthiasis) in Lubumbashi. Santé Publique;**15**(4):413-421

[41] Njeru A, Mutuku F, Muriu S. Status of soil-transmitted helminthiasis among pregnant women attending antenatal clinic in Kilifi county hospital, Kenya. bioRxiv. 2019;**1**:613570

[42] Hillier SD, Booth M, Muhangi L, Nkurunziza P, Khihembo M, Kakande M, et al. *Plasmodium falciparum* and helminth coinfection in a semiurban population of pregnant women in Uganda. The Journal of Infectious Diseases. 2008;**198**(6):920-927

[43] Ndibazza J, Webb EL, Lule S, Mpairwe H, Akello M, Oduru G, et al. Associations between maternal helminth and malaria infections in pregnancy and clinical malaria in the offspring: A birth cohort in Entebbe, Uganda. The Journal of Infectious Diseases. 2013;**208**(12):2007-2016

[44] Geophagy: "Soil-Eating" as an Addictive Behaviour. ScienceDaily. 2019. Available from: https://www.sciencedaily.com/releases/2016/12/161205085943.htm

[45] Kawai K, Saathoff E, Antelman G, Msamanga G, Fawzi WW. Geophagy (soil-eating) in relation to anemia and

helminth infection among HIV–Infected pregnant women in Tanzania. The American Journal of Tropical Medicine and Hygiene. 2009;**80**(1):36-43

[46] Luoba AI, Geissler PW, Estambale B, Ouma JH, Alusala D, Ayah R, et al. Earth-eating and reinfection with intestinal helminths among pregnant and lactating women in western Kenya. Tropical Medicine and International Health. 2005;**10**(3):220-227

[47] Larocque R, Casapia M, Gotuzzo E, Gyorkos TW. Relationship between intensity of soil-transmitted helminth infections and anemia during pregnancy. The American Journal of Tropical Medicine and Hygiene. 2005;**73**(4):783-789

[48] Fuseinisup G, Edohsup D, Kalifasup BG, Hamidsup A-W, Knight D. Parasitic infections and anaemia during pregnancy in the Kassena-Nankana district of Northern Ghana. JPHE. 2010;**2**(3):48-52

[49] Gyorkos TW, Gilbert NL, Larocque R, Casapía M. Trichuris and hookworm infections associated with anaemia during pregnancy. Tropical Medicine & International Health. 2011;**16**(4):531-537

[50] Naing C, Whittaker MA, Nyunt-Wai V, Reid SA, Wong SF, Mak JW, et al. Malaria and soil-transmitted intestinal helminth co-infection and its effect on anemia: A meta-analysis. Transactions of the Royal Society of Tropical Medicine and Hygiene. 2013;**107**(11):672-683

[51] Bánhidy F, Ács N, Puhó EH, Czeizel AE. Iron deficiency anemia: Pregnancy outcomes with or without iron supplementation. Nutrition. 2011;**27**(1):65-72

[52] Eiríksdóttir VH, Ásgeirsdóttir TL, Bjarnadóttir RI, Kaestner R, Cnattingius S, Valdimarsdóttir UA. Low birth weight, small for gestational age and preterm births before and after the economic collapse in Iceland: A population based cohort study. PLoS One. 2013;**8**(12):e80499

[53] Passerini L, Casey GJ, Biggs BA, Cong DT, Phu LB, Phuc TQ, et al. Increased birth weight associated with regular pre-pregnancy deworming and weekly iron-folic acid supplementation for Vietnamese women. PLoS Neglected Tropical Diseases. 2012;**6**(4):e1608

[54] McSorley HJ, Maizels RM. Helminth infections and host immune regulation. Clinical Microbiology Reviews. 2012;**25**(4):585-608

[55] Weinstock JV, Elliott DE. Helminths and the IBD hygiene hypothesis. Inflammatory Bowel Diseases. 2009;**15**(1):128-133

[56] Fusunyan RD, Sanderson IR. Inflammatory bowel disease. In: Delves PJ, editor. Encyclopedia of Immunology. 2nd ed. Oxford: Elsevier; 1998. pp. 1375-1381. Available from: http://www.sciencedirect.com/science/article/pii/B0122267656003625

[57] Moskaluk CA. Esophagus. In: Weidner N, Cote RJ, Suster S, Weiss LM, editors. Modern Surgical Pathology. 2nd ed. Philadelphia: W.B. Saunders; 2009. pp. 637-672. Available from: http://www.sciencedirect.com/science/article/pii/B9781416039662000205

[58] Elliott DE, Urban JF, Argo CK, Weinstock JV. Does the failure to acquire helminthic parasites predispose to Crohn's disease? The FASEB Journal. 2000;**14**(12):1848-1855

[59] Wiria AE, Hamid F, Wammes LJ, Prasetyani MA, Dekkers OM, May L, et al. Infection with soil-transmitted helminths is associated with increased insulin sensitivity. PLoS One. 2015;**10**(6):e0127746

[60] Hotez P. Hookworm and poverty. Annals of the New York Academy of Sciences. 2008;**1136**(1):38-44

[61] Holland CV, Taren DL, Crompton DWT, Nesheim MC, Sanjur D, Barbeau I, et al. Intestinal helminthiases in relation to the socioeconomic environment of Panamanian children. Social Science and Medicine. 1988;**26**(2):209-213

[62] Raso G, Utzinger J, Silué KD, Ouattara M, Yapi A, Toty A, et al. Disparities in parasitic infections, perceived ill health and access to health care among poorer and less poor schoolchildren of rural Côte d'Ivoire. Tropical Medicine and International Health. 2005;**10**(1):42-57

[63] Olsen A, Samuelsen H, Onyango-Ouma W. A study of risk factors for intestinal helminth infections using epidemiological and anthropological approaches. Journal of Biosocial Science. 2001;**33**(4):569-584

Chapter 3

Soil-Transmitted Helminths

Richard R. Roach

Abstract

Helminths currently affect over 2 billion people worldwide with a quarter of the world's population infected at some time in their lives. Sobering statistics from the WHO March 2008 report that 80% of the "Bottom Billion" impoverished population of the world have *Ascaris*, 60% have *Trichuris*, and 57% have hookworms. This would only be a problem of pharmacologic distribution if not for an additional report demonstrating that several new studies reported to the WHO claim a 50% failure rate clearing *Trichuris* and 90% failure rate clearing hookworm. These parasitic infections pose a challenge to tropical physicians who have considered mebendazole and albendazole as adequate treatments for children. This is even more of a challenge for physicians in temperate climates who may be less familiar with these medications. This article presents the recent data and the approach to treatment failure and new therapeutic approaches.

Keywords: helminths, *Ascaris*, *Trichuris*, hookworm

1. Introduction

Intestinal parasites cause substantial morbidity and mortality, particularly in children in whom they have detrimental effects on growth and cognitive performance. Parasitic infestation leads to deformity and long-term disabilities and often stigmatizes the child. Parasitized pregnant women are anemic, have increased fetal wastage, and have low birth weight newborns. Though tropical diseases affect a large proportion of the world's population, less than 1% of new drug development over the past 30 years focused on tropical diseases. Recent philanthropic interest has resulted in research, long tardy, for these diseases.

2. Epidemiology

There are three soil-transmitted helminth infections, *Ascaris lumbricoides*, hookworm (*Ancylostoma duodenale* and *Necator americanus*), and *Trichuris trichiura*, labeled by the WHO as the "Unholy Trinity." They are ubiquitous in tropical climates and even temperate rural areas in poverty-stricken communities with poor sanitation (see **Table 1**). *Ascaris* and *Trichuris* increase in prevalence from infancy to puberty and then decrease in adulthood. In contrast, hookworm, the leading cause of anemia throughout the world, continues to increase through life, not reaching a plateau until age 40. This characteristic has a profound effect on women of childbearing age and is associated with small-for-gestation newborns as well as increasing fetal loss.

Disease	Global prevalence (millions) [1]	Population at risk (billions)	Estimated global disease burden (disability-adjusted life years in millions)	Vulnerable population
Ascariasis	807	4.2	1.8–10.5	School-age children
Trichuriasis	604	3.2	1.8–6.4	School-age children
Hookworm	576	3.2	1.5–22.1	School-age children, women of reproductive age

Table 1.
Impact of soil-transmitted helminths [2].

3. Management

The WHO has classified parasitic infestation by egg intensity to clarify symptomatic and asymptomatic infestations (see **Table 2**). Children with light worm loads are often asymptomatic, but children form the greatest population of the heavy intensity group. Even children considered asymptomatic may have subtle differences in learning and intellectual achievement [1].

The clinical presentation relates to parasite migration in the skin, viscera, and gastrointestinal tract. *Trichuris* and *Ascaris* are a result of fecal-oral ingestion. Wheezing, dyspnea, nonproductive cough, fever, bloody sputum, chest x-ray infiltrates, and systemic eosinophilia result during pulmonary vascular migration. Once swallowed the larvae mature, and their migration in the gut causes abdominal pain, distention, and malabsorption.

If adult *Ascaris* migrate into the biliary tree, then pancreatitis, cholangitis, and cholecystitis result. Hepatic abscesses and appendicitis may result from *Ascaris* migration. In younger children, heavy loads of worms can cause partial or complete bowel obstruction in the ileum. Swelling of Peyer's patches leads to an increased risk of intussusception and volvulus. Unrecognized obstruction may eventually cause bowel infarction and perforation with resulting peritonitis.

Trichuris may infect any part of the colon, but the parasite prefers the cecum. Eggs release the larvae in the small intestine, and the worms mature in the colon where they tunnel into the mucosa, causing inflammation. Heavy infestation causes a dysentery syndrome severe enough that it may result in rectal prolapse. Impaired growth and anemia are the consequences of chronic infestation.

Hookworm infects through skin penetration. Itching erythematous rash from multiple skin penetrations causes severe pruritus of the skin, usually on the feet or hands. The larvae use the pulmonary vasculature to access the bronchial secretions and then, when swallowed, mature into adults in the gastrointestinal tract. Bronchial migration presents as clinical pneumonitis but may be mistaken for asthma. Pulmonary symptoms are seldom as dramatic as with *Ascaris*. The significant sequelae of infection relate to intestinal blood loss. As few as 40 worms can reduce the hemoglobin below 11 g/dl. Heavy infestations lead to loss of protein with resulting loss of plasma osmotic pressure and anasarca.

Helminth infestations cause anemia and malnutrition, growth stunting, and cognitive deficits, associated with poor school attendance and performance. Since this occurs in an impoverished area where the diet has limited resource to protein, the consequences of the poor child's limited diet magnifies the malnutrition. If this occurs in a malaria area, the anemia caused by helminths exaggerates the anemia of malaria.

Intensity	*Ascaris*	*Hookworms*	*Trichuris*
Light	1–4999 epg	1–1999 epg	1–999 epg
Moderate	5000–49,999 epg	2000–3999 epg	1000–9999 epg
Heavy	≥50,000 epg	≥4000 epg	≥10,000 epg

Epg: eggs per gram of feces.

Table 2.
Soil-transmitted helminth infection intensity [3].

This is especially crucial for women of childbearing age, since infected women were 2.6 times more likely to have preterm deliveries and 3.5 times more likely to have small-for-gestational age infants. If the woman lives in a malaria-endemic area, the risks of malaria increase the infant mortality.

4. Treatment

There are four medications currently available to treat soil-transmitted helminth infections (see **Table 3**). Benzimidazoles impede the microtubular system, in particular β-tubulin, in the worm. Since this is not a host system, patients tolerate these drugs with minimal side effects. Very few patients report nausea, vomiting, and headache, but allergic reactions with fever are rare. Levamisole and pyrantel pamoate are nicotinic acetylcholine receptor agonists, which paralyze the worms and precipitate their expulsion. Gastrointestinal symptoms, headache, dizziness, fever, and rash are usually mild and self-limited. However, a bulk of paralyzed worms increases the risk of a bowel obstruction.

The most important aspect of treatment is efficacy. Cure rates and egg reduction rates are high for all four drugs when treating *Ascaris* (see **Table 4**). Nevertheless, recent studies have documented ineffective and inconsistent treatment of *Trichuris* and hookworm, whether *Ancylostoma duodenale* or *Necator americanus*. The concern is drug resistance, despite lack of previous investigation. Researchers presumed that the drugs were effective in the past because they were effective with the other

Infection	Drug	Dose
Ascariasis	Albendazole*	400 mg once
	Mebendazole	100 mg twice daily × 3 days or 500 mg once
	Pyrantel pamoate	11 mg/kg (max 1 g) × 3 days
	Levamisole	2.5 mg/kg once
Hookworm	Albendazole*	400 mg once
	Mebendazole	100 mg twice daily × 3 days
	Pyrantel pamoate	11 mg/kg (max 1 g) × 3 days
	Levamisole	2.5 mg/kg once, repeat after 7 days for heavy infection
Trichuris	Mebendazole	100 mg twice daily × 3 days or 500 mg once
	Albendazole*	400 mg × 3 days

**In children 1–2 years old, use 200 mg.*

Table 3.
Treatment of soil-transmitted helminth infections [6].

Parasite	Drug	Dose	Cure rate (%)	Egg reduction rate (%)
A. lumbricoides	Albendazole	400 mg once	88[a,b]	87–100[a]
	Mebendazole	500 mg once	95[a,b]	96–100[a]
		100 mg twice a day for 3 days	92[c]	91–100[c]
	Pyrantel pamoate	10 mg/kg once	88[a,b]	88[a]
		10 mg/kg for 3 days	92[d]	99[d]
	Levamisole	2.5 mg/kg once	92[a]	92–100[a]
Hookworm	Albendazole	400 mg once	72[a,b]	64–100[a]
	Mebendazole	500 mg once	15[a,b]	0–98[a]
		100 mg twice a day for 3 days	80[e]	41–100[e]
	Pyrantel pamoate	10 mg/kg once	31[a,b]	56–75[a]
		10 mg/kg for 3 days	68[d]	77–99[d]
	Levamisole	2.5 mg/kg once	38[a]	68–100[a]
T. trichiura	Albendazole	400 mg once	28[a,b]	0–90[a]
	Albendazole	400 mg for 3 days	53[f]	81–100[f]
	Mebendazole	500 mg once	36[a,b]	81–93[a]
		100 mg twice a day for 3 days	63[g]/ 80[h]	38–99[g]
	Pyrantel pamoate	10 mg/kg once	31[a]	52[a]
		10 mg/kg for 3 days	27[d]	77[d]
	Levamisole	2.5 mg/kg once	10[a]	42[a]
S. stercoralis	Ivermectin	200 μg/kg once	88[i]	N/A
	Ivermectin	200 μg/kg for 2 days	96[j]	N/A
	Albendazole	400 mg once	69[k]	N/A
	Albendazole	400 mg twice daily for 3 days	62[k]	N/A

N/A, not applicable.
[a] Data derived from recent systematic review and meta-analysis (Keiser and Utzinger, 2008).
[b] Data from randomised controlled trials.
[c] Overall cure rate and egg reduction rates based on 29 trials.
[d] Overall cure rate and egg reduction rates based on three trials (Botero and Castano, 1973; Kale et al., 1982; Seah, 1973).
[e] Overall cure rate and egg reduction rates based on 27 trials.
[f] Overall cure rate and egg reduction rates based on five trials (Adams et al., 2004; Marti et al., 1996; Okelo, 1984; Sirivichayakul et al., 2001; Zhang et al., 1990).
[g] Overall cure rate and egg reduction rates based on 33 trials.
[h] Combined pooled relative risk of four randomised controlled trials (Davison, 1979; Sargent et al., 1975; Vandepitte et al., 1973; Wesche and Barnish, 1994).
[i] Overall cure rate based on six trials (Datry et al., 1994; Gann et al., 1994; Igual-Adell et al., 2004; Marti et al., 1996; Shikiya et al., 1991b, 1992).
[j] Overall cure rate based on three trials (Gann et al., 1994; Igual-Adell et al., 2004; Ordonez and Angulo, 2004).
[k] Based on literature review by Horton (2000).

Table 4.
Efficacy of single- and multiple-dose anthelminthic drugs against common soil-transmitted helminth infections [4].

helminths. Recent studies by veterinarians tested efficacy in mass drug administration to animals in endemic areas. Such studies presumed human efficacy. Subsequent studies done in adults excluded children and pregnant women, the most at-risk populations.

Currently, research established benzimidazoles as safe for children greater than 1 year of age. Teratogenic potential seen in animal studies requires careful assessment of benefit/risk ratio. The WHO does recommend treatment of hookworm in pregnancy due to the adverse effect of anemia which is greater than the risk of the medication [2]. Limited studies show no congenital anomalies or perinatal mortality with the use of albendazole, mebendazole, or ivermectin, although use in the first trimester is still discouraged. Studies have yet to focus on levamisole and pyrantel in pregnancy [2].

5. Prevention

Because of the large burden of disease, prevention needs to be the foremost consideration in improving community health. Sanitation, access to a clean source of water, and careful food preparation limit fecal-oral contamination. Careful disposal of feces decreases exposure to helminthic eggs, and footwear limits hookworm exposure.

The other approach has been to limit morbidity through periodic treatment. The school system has been the logical institution for community treatment. Many studies have employed deworming schoolchildren on an annual basis, while others have focused on women of reproductive age. One recent study focused on community versus schoolchildren treatment justified a strategy that involves the entire community [3]. Community treatment in several studies documents the requirement to reach at least 75% of the at-risk population. Governments willing to institute such programs recognize the cost of $0.02 USD. Several pharmaceutical companies made the drugs affordable. One example, a study done in Zanzibar, examined the co-administration of ivermectin, albendazole, and praziquantel in 5055 children and adults. This mass drug administration benefitted the entire community.

6. Future research and treatment

Considering the high prevalence of soil-transmitted helminths and the established resistance, there is a need for other treatment options. This has provoked enthusiasm for vaccines and drugs with novel mechanisms of action. Unfortunately, there has been little financial incentive for developing human vaccines and novel drugs for poverty-stricken areas, but veterinary medicine has the financial incentive of herd treatment.

The nicotinic acetylcholine receptor is unique to helminths and nematodes, although it appears to be a malaria parasite receptor as well. Since this receptor does not exist in humans, a medication to block this receptor should be effective and well tolerated. A vaccine with an antibody against this receptor seems a logical potential step for research. Tribendimidine is an L-type nicotinic acetylcholine receptor agonist. It is very effective in animals. Clinical trial in humans resulted in approval in China in 2004. Despite the difference in chemical structure and the hypothesized receptor agonist effect, it proved to have the same mechanism of action as benzimidazoles and showed no advantage in humans.

Monepantel is a nicotinic acetylcholine receptor agonist. It is highly effective and licensed for sheep. Researchers initiated studies in humans. It does appear to have a unique mechanism of action since in animals it has been effective in multidrug resistant nematode infections it may also be effective in humans with resistant infestations.

Developing a vaccine requires an antigen. Developers have struggled with which antigen to use that will allow a sufficient and effective antigenic response. Vaccines developed for soil-transmitted helminths are effective in newborn animals. A vaccine to the hookworm antigen, Na-ASP-2, is effective in dogs [4]. Vaccinated while still puppies, they were resistant to hookworm infection. This success led to a limited phase 1 trial in Brazil. Unfortunately, 30% of the patients developed urticaria, and one patient developed anaphylaxis. These reactions stopped the trial. Speculation as to the cause of this intense reaction led to the hypothesis that the study patients had antibodies to the antigen because of previous exposure from residing in an endemic area. Like the puppies, the requirement must to vaccinate human subjects prior to antigenic exposure [5].

7. Conclusions

Helminth infections are a common problem. Presumed effectiveness of drugs is a deficient hypothesis. The available medications are not as effective as once thought. The trials of mass treatment of schoolchildren do not exterminate the source of infection or resolve the community exposure. New medication research is essential, especially for *Trichuris*. Novel treatments such as vaccines may be on the horizon, but safety concerns for humans with previous exposure is an important immunologic problem. Sanitation is still the most important community solution. The recent disaster in Port-au-Prince, Haiti, demonstrated that without sewer systems and potable water, we humans are indeed a vulnerable species.

Author details

Richard R. Roach
Internal Medicine Department, Western Michigan University School of Medicine, Kalamazoo, MI, USA

*Address all correspondence to: richard.roach@med.wmich.edu

References

[1] Hotez PJ, Molyneux DH, Fenwick A, Kumaresan J, Sachs SE, Sachs JD, et al. Control of neglected tropical diseases. The New England Journal of Medicine. 2007;**357**(10):1018-1027

[2] Allen HE, Crompton DW, de Silva N, LoVerde PT, Olds GR. New policies for using anthelmintics in high risk groups. Trends in Parasitology. 2002;**18**(9):381-382. DOI: 10.1016/S1471-4922(02)02386-3

[3] Pullan RL, Halliday KE, Oswald WE, Ncgari C, et al. Effects, equity, and cost of school-based and community-wide treatment strategies for soil-transmitted helminths in Kenya: A cluster-randomised controlled trial. The Lancet. 2019;**393**(10185):2039-2050

[4] Keiser J, Utzinger J. The drugs we have and the drugs we need against major helminth infections. In: Xiao-Nong Zhou RBRO, Jürg U, editors. Advances in Parasitology. Vol. 73. Academic Press; 2010. pp. 197-230

[5] Lemoine JF, Desormeaux AM, Monestime F, Fayette CR, et al. Controlling neglected tropical diseases in Haiti: Implementation strategies and evidence of their success. PLOS Neglected Tropical Diseases. 2016;**10**(10):e0004954

[6] Muchiri EM, et al. A comparative study of different albendazole and mebendazole regimens for the treatment of intestinal infections in school children of Usigu Division, western Kenya. Journal of Parasitology. 2001;**87**(2):413-418

Section 3

Nematodes Infections

Chapter 4

Filariasis

Sharba Kausar

Abstract

Filariasis is one of the most debilitating tropical neglected diseases with high morbidity rate and less rate of mortality with various clinical symptoms. According to the World Health Organization (WHO) reports, about 120 million people from 81 countries are infected at present, and an estimated 1.34 billion people live in areas endemic to filariasis and are at risk of infection. Currently available drugs are only effective against the larval stage of the worms with side effects, and their repetitive use gives rise to drug resistance. Till date, no effective vaccine is available for the treatment of filariasis; to fulfill this need, new drug development becomes the priority for the researchers. This chapter reviews different synthetic and natural origin drugs, drug targets, and use of bioinformatics to discover new antifilarial agents which can control this debilitating disease, including the types of filariasis, their prevalence, and eradication programs which are discussed.

Keywords: filariasis, drug targets, antifilarials, bioinformatics

1. Introduction

A variety of parasitic diseases which are associated with morbidity and mortality have received less attention worldwide. Among these, filariasis is one of the most debilitating neglected tropical diseases. Filariasis is a vector-borne disease transmitted by arthropod vector which is endemic in the tropics and subtropics that results in social stigma. It is a group of human and animal infectious diseases caused by nematode parasites generally called "filariae" that include several hundred species of worms that are slender and elongated and are parasitic in tissues of various vertebrate hosts. This parasite known to cause human infections belongs mainly to the genera *Wuchereria*, *Brugia*, *Onchocerca*, *Dipetalonema*, *Mansonella*, and *Loa*. They reside either in lymphatics or muscles, connective tissues, body cavities, etc. of vertebrate hosts. They may be classified into three main groups based on the habitat of the adult worm, i.e., the cutaneous group, the lymphatic group, and the body cavity group. Based on the habitat of the adult worm, a few of the filarial species infecting man and the disease caused by them with their intermediate hosts are listed in **Table 1**. The infection is transmitted by intermediate hosts which are always blood-sucking arthropods of the order Diptera. Only two genera, *Wuchereria* and *Brugia*, are mainly responsible for human lymphatic filariasis. The common animal parasites are *Setaria digitata* and *S. cervi* (bovine), *Dirofilaria immitis* (dog), *D. uniformis* (rabbit), *Litomosoides carinii* and *Dipetalonema vitae* (gerbils), *Brugia pahangi* (cat), and *Acanthocheilonema viteae* (jird).

According to recent surveys, about 120 million people in 81 countries of the world are infected from this disease, and 1.34 billion people who live in endemic areas are at high risk of this life-threatening infection [1]. To eradicate filariasis

IntechOpen

Filarial worm	Habitat	Intermediate host	Disease
Wuchereria bancrofti	Lymphatics	Mosquito sp.	Elephantiasis
Brugia malayi	Lymphatics	Mosquito sp.	Malayan filariasis
B. timori	Lymphatics	Mosquito sp.	Timor fever
Loa loa	Connective tissue	*Chrysopsis* sp. (*C. dimidiata*)—Horse flies	Loaiasis
Mansonella ozzardi	Serous membranes	*Culicoides* sp. (*C. furens*)—biting midges	Ozzard's filaria
Onchocerca volvulus	Skin	*Simulium* sp. (*S. damnosum*)—black flies	Onchocerciasis

Table 1.
List of filarial worms with their habitats and intermediate host infecting humans.

globally, research plans are needed to design effective drugs and drug targets, new vector control strategies, and diagnostic techniques. At the same time, the treatment of filariasis also requires disease-specific clinical care and patient education with counseling to eradicate this disease. Moreover, statistical analysis along with bioinformatics tools of the mass drug administration (MDA) surveillance reports should be carried out which could provide new opportunities to get an insight into the proteins or genome which may contribute to its inhibition process.

In current surveillance report, five World Health Organization (WHO) regions are endemic with lymphatic filariasis (LF). Worldwide, 1.39 billion people require preventive chemotherapy. In Southeast Asia region, 877 million people of 9 countries and 432 million people of 39 countries in the Africa region are brutally affected from this disease and require proper treatment. From the Western Pacific Region which includes the Mekong Plus region and the Pacific region, nearly 40 million people are at a risk of lymphatic filariasis. Cambodia, China, Cook Islands, Niue, the Marshall Islands, Palau, the Republic of Korea, Tonga, Vanuatu, Viet Nam, and Wallis and Futuna are the countries of this region that successfully eradicated this disease, whereas American Samoa, Brunei Darussalam, Fiji, French Polynesia, Kiribati, Lao People's Democratic Republic, Malaysia, Federated States of Micronesia, New Caledonia, Papua New Guinea, Philippines, Samoa and Tuvalu are the 13 countries where lymphatic filariasis remains endemic [1, 2].

2. History of filariasis

In India first, ancient documented evidence of filariasis was reported in *Sushruta Samhita* (approximately 600 BC) by the famous physician Sushruta. According to some records, the first reliable documentation of filariasis was reported in the late fifteenth and early sixteenth centuries. In 1849 William Prout explained the pathological condition of chyluria in which the passage of lymph occurs in urine, a condition associated with lymphatic filariasis. The French surgeon Jean Nicolas in 1863 was the first person who observed the microfilariae in the hydrocele fluid. For the first time, in 1872 Timothy Lewis observed the microfilariae in the human blood in India. In 1876, Joseph Bancroft recovered female filarial worms and named them *Filaria bancrofti*, which later merged in the genus *Wuchereria*. In 1877, Sir Patrick Manson discovered the main cause of transmission of filariasis, by studying the parasitic development of microfilariae in the mosquito stomach that was fed on the blood of an infected gardener and thus reported that filariasis is transmitted by the mosquito. In 1960 and 1977, two other filarial worm species were identified and named as *Brugia malayi* and *B. timori*, respectively.

3. Filariasis: an overview

Among all the filariasis, lymphatic filariasis is the most debilitating which causes disability in humans. *Wuchereria bancrofti* and *Brugia malayi* or *B. timori* are the main cause of lymphatic filariasis, each of which is transmitted by the bite of a specific insect vector. The various vectors that cause LF belong to the genera *Anopheles*, *Culex*, *Aedes*, and *Mansonia*. According to the WHO, increase in the microfilarial density in the infected individuals and the feeding rate of vector population are the causes of high transmission rates of filariasis in a particular area. *Onchocerca volvulus* and *Loa loa* are the two other filarial worms that reside in the cutaneous and subcutaneous tissues of the host and cause onchocerciasis and loaiasis, respectively. *Wuchereria bancrofti* and *O. volvulus* are the two filarial worms which do not require an animal host as reservoir.

Data collected from the survey depicted the picture of depressive illness of an individual caused by LF and estimated 5.09 million disability-adjusted life years (DALYs) [3–5]. In infants microfilaremia starts at the age of 5 after acquiring infection, but the actual signs of filariasis (including hydroceles) appear during puberty. Previous survey reports indicated that once the individual acquired infection chances of cure becomes very low [6].

Filarial worms inhabiting the lymphatic system live up to 8 years and release millions of microfilariae into the bloodstream. The WHO started the Global Alliance to Eliminate Lymphatic Filariasis (GPELF) in 2000 with the goal of eradicating this disease by 2020 through the use of MDA [7]. In the history of public health, GPELF is the most successfully expanding global health program. Fifty-three out of the 81 endemic countries have started mass drug administration to halt the transmission of filariasis. Two strategies have been developed to achieve the target of eliminating filariasis. According to the first strategy, single annual doses of diethylcarbamazine or ivermectin plus albendazole will be provided to the entire endemic area to prevent the disease. The second strategy is to reduce disability rate by providing knowledge about how to maintain hygiene and skin care, to those with lymphedema and performing surgery in patients with hydrocele. The investment for chemotherapy to control this disease is approximately US$ 105–208 million per year during 2015–2020. The WHO determined two objectives, which include "70% of endemic countries demanding MDA will have to enter post-intervention surveillance by 2016" and "all other endemic countries have to complete the post-intervention surveillance by 2020" [8, 9]. The abovementioned antifilarial drugs are only effective against the microfilariae and have no effect on the adult worms which therefore provide a partial treatment to the infected individuals. Repetitive use of these drugs resulted in drug resistance. Till date no vaccines are developed, and treatment depends only on the antifilarial. Researchers are developing various new antifilarials and combination therapies to overcome this disease [10].

4. General life cycle of filarial worm

Man is the definitive host of filarial worm, in whose lymphatic system, the adult worms reside. Adult females discharge the live embryo called microfilariae (290 μ). Microfilariae flow in the peripheral blood and can survive for a considerable time

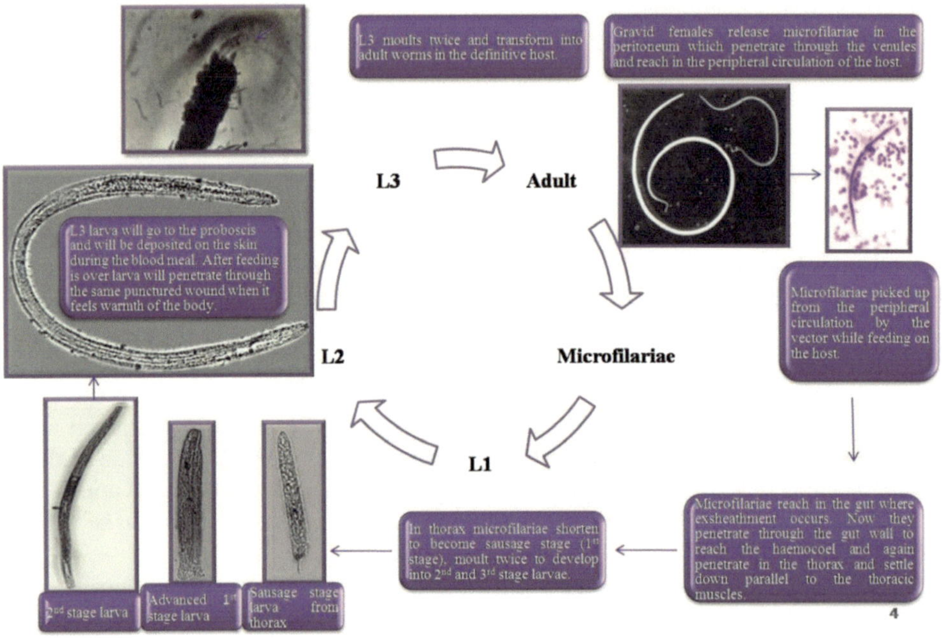

Figure 1.
Life cycle of filarial worm Setaria cervi *given by Prof. Wajihullah and Dr. Sharba Kausar.*

without undergoing metamorphosis until they are taken up by the intermediate host, i.e., the culicine mosquitoes during their blood meal. After reaching in the mosquitoes, microfilariae undergo development and become infective-stage larvae as described in **Figure 1**.

5. Diagnosis of lymphatic filariasis

LF is primarily diagnosed using the immunochromatographic card test kit via antigen detection methods (which also detects latent infections). The traditional diagnosis of LF is performed by microscopy to detect circulating microfilariae. Molecular xenomonitoring of parasites in mosquitoes, serological testing, ultrasonography, PCR tests, lymphoscintigraphy, detection of exposure to transmission in children via antibody detection, and the recently introduced filariasis test strip (FTS) are some of the other diagnostic approaches that are currently used.

6. Biological point for designing new drug

A clear knowledge of parasite physiology is very important to identify drug targets for understanding the mode of action of antifilarial drug. Sometimes compounds are also tested, without prior knowledge of the target. Compounds which are effective against the whole parasite are defined as hits, while compounds that are found to be active in vivo are considered as leads. Lead compounds require standardization for increasing their efficacy. Once a compound is optimized, it can be tested clinically in patients and defined as a "drug candidate." Based on the physiological processes and symptoms, a drug should be formulated and designed to combat the disease. To overcome filariasis a number of drug targets should be covered for developing new antifilarial, viz., macrofilaricidal and microfilaricidal drugs, drugs preventing exsheathment in microfilariae and drugs that can cause hindrance in the movement of microfilariae. Different biochemical pathways are summarized in **Table 2** which are used in designing new drugs. On the other hand,

***Wolbachia* bacteria**		
Wolbachia are proteobacteria 61 potential drug targets (outer membrane proteins, ribosomal proteins, DNA polymerases, mutases, ligases, isomerases, cell division proteins, transferases, synthetases, reductases, etc.) and four potential vaccine extracellular targets such as putative peptidoglycan lipid II flippase, deoxycytidine triphosphate deaminase, GTP cyclohydrolase II, and RNA pyrophosphohydrolase	Contribute to the nucleotide pool of nematodes	Tetracycline was resulted in the depletion of these *Wolbachia* resulting in the upregulation of phosphate permease gene, required for nucleotide synthesis Another study with doxycycline showed that *Wolbachia* depletion was associated with a reduction in the levels of vascular endothelial growth factors (VEGFs) that are essential for lymphangiogenesis (18)
Wolbachia cell division protein FtsZ a GTPase	Bacteria-specific filamenting temperature-sensitive protein (important in bacterial cytokinesis) that was expressed in all developmental stages of *B. malayi*	*E. coli* FtsZ inhibitor berberine, a natural alkaloid, was examined by researchers against GTPase activity of FtsZ in *B. malayi*, and it was observed that at 10–40 mM concentration, berberine had adversely affected production of microfilariae as well as motility of adult females of *B. malayi*
N-Myristoyltransferase		
Myristoyltransferase (NMT)	The addition of myristic acid, a 14-carbon unsaturated fatty acid, to the N-terminus of glycine in a subset of proteins via myristoyl-CoA:protein N-myristoyltransferase (NMT) promotes their binding to cell membrane	A known NMT enzyme inhibitor in tripanosomatids, DDD85646, and its analog DDD100870, were tested against *B. malayi* NMT proteins and provided IC50 values of 10 nM and 2.5 nM, respectively
Proteins and amino acids		
	Free amino acids are required for intracellular osmoregulation and protein synthesis	
S-adenosylmethionine methyltransferase, methionine adenosyltransferase, and S-adenosylhomocysteine hydrolase	Are required for the conversion of methionine to homocysteine in the methionine	
Enzyme prolyl-4-hydroxylase has been reported to	Play a vital role in the biosynthesis of this collagen	
Transaminoglutamase	Play a significant role in the growth, development, and maturation of the nematode	A pseudosubstrate, monodansylcadaverine (MDC), and active site inhibitors cystamine or iodoacetamide were found to inhibit L3-stage parasite mobility in a dose-dependent manner that was associated with irreversible biochemical lesions, resulting in the death of the parasite

Proteins and amino acids		
Retinoic acid-binding proteins (RABPs)	Parasitic nematodes require lipophilic retinol for various biological processes, such as embryogenesis, differentiation, and growth For inter- as well as intracellular movement	Ivermectin(II) was found to compete efficiently with retinol for the retinol-binding sites on RBP of the parasite but not for the host RBP sites
Biogenic amines and polyamines		
Norepinephrine (NE), histamine, 5-hydroxytryptamine (5-HT), and dopamine	Biogenic amines play a role in neuromuscular activity and behavioral coordination in nematodes	
Monoamine oxidase (i.e., MAO), acetylcholinesterase, and dopamine-b-hydroxylase		DEC, levamisole, and centperazine were found to inactivate these enzymes
Dopamine-b-hydroxylase		
Octopamine		
Putrescine, spermine, and spermidine	Are required for growth, differentiation, and macromolecular synthesis in all living organisms as constituents of the polyamine salvage pathway	
S-adenosylmethionine decarboxylase (SAMDC)	Which is required for polyamine biosynthesis	Berenil and aromatic methylglyoxal bis (guanylhydrazone) analogs are inhibitors of an important regulatory enzyme
Carbohydrate metabolism		
Fructose 1,6-diphosphate aldolase	Its immunogenic component in filarial worms is distinguishable from that of mammals, thus identifying it as possible vaccine target238	
Phosphoenolpyruvate carboxykinase	Inhibited by DEC	
Fumarate reductase	Inhibited by DEC and benzimidazoles	
Succinate dehydrogenase	Inhibited by DEC	
Phosphofructokinase	Blocked by antimonial stibophen in *B. pahangi* and *L. carinii* when compared to isofunctional mammalian enzyme	
Glucose uptake	Altered by DEC, amoscanate, and arsenicals	
Utilization of glucose	Decreased by levamisole	
Lipid metabolism		
Quinones	Play a role in filarial electron transport	
Geranyl geraniol	Unknown role	The biosynthesis of genanyl geraniol and dolichols was inhibited by mevinolin

Lipid metabolism		
Juvenile hormones	Regulators of larval development	
Dolichols	Required for glycoprotein synthesis	
Isopentyl pyrophosphate	IPP constituent of filarial tRNA	
HMG-CoA reductase is a rate limiting enzyme	Involved in the isoprenoid pathway of filaria	Inhibited by mevinolin
Folate metabolism		
Enzymes, such as reductases, transferases, synthases, dehydrogenases, hydrolases, mutases, ligases, and deaminases	Are involved in the interconversation of folate analogs observed in the synthesis of different tetrahydrofolate cofactors by macrofilariae. Specifically, dihydrofolate reductase activity, which is commonly observed in macrofilariae, was found to be absent in the microfilariae of *B. pahangi*	DEC and suramin were found to inhibit some enzymes involved in folate metabolism
10-Formyl FH4 dehydrogenase enzyme	Which was found to play a vital role in the regulation of the endogenous FH4 cofactor concentrations, was more active in *B. pahangi* than in mammals	
Glutathione		
Glutamate-cysteine ligase (rate-g-glutamyl transpeptidase)	Glutathione has been proposed to constitute the antioxidant system (g-glutamyl cycle) that extends the survival of filarial parasites in mammalian hosts, thereby protecting them from host-mediated membrane lipid peroxidation	Arsenicals depletes filarial glutathione (262–264) Phytocompounds such as plumbagin, curcumin, and a phenoxyacetic acid derivative were found to inhibit filarial GST In a report of a homology modeling approach via in silico analysis of the filarial GST of *B. malayi*, albendazole, and a methyl-substituted chalcone showed non-competitive type of inhibition of GST activity
Glutathione-transferases (GSTs)	The major detoxifying systems in filarial parasites and can detoxify cytotoxic products of lipid peroxidation via the conjugation of glutathione (GSH) to various endogenous xenobiotic electrophiles	

Table 2.
Antifilarial targets for designing drugs.

vaccine development and mosquito repellent practices such as the use of insecticide nets, body lotions, insecticides spray, coils, etc. along with good knowledge of sanitization can prevent vector development which together helps in combating filarial worm infection in a community. The pathology associated with lymphatic filariasis like elephantiasis, hydrocoele, and lymphedema is due to the hyporesponsiveness of D4+ T cells of the host immune system [11–13]. Therefore, immunological studies are also playing an important role in the field of drug development. Drugs are also designed to combat symptoms associated with filariasis, viz., drugs used for the treatment of lymphatic filariasis (drugs effective against adenolymphadenitis, funiculitis, epididymo-orchitis, lymphedema, hydrocele, chyluria, chylocele, lymph scrotum) and drugs used in the treatment of other manifestations like asymptomatic microfilaremia, occult filariasis, onchocerciasis, and loaiasis.

7. Currently used antifilarial drugs

7.1 Diethylcarbamazine (DEC)

Diethylcarbamazine (DEC), a piperazine derivative, is the most common and widely used drug over many decades. The antifilarial activity of DEC was first tested against *Litomosoides carinii*- and *Dirofilaria immitis*-infected cotton rats and dogs, respectively [8]. The observations revealed DEC as a potential microfilaricidal agent. Clinical trial of DEC was started in 1947 against human filariasis. Later, strong antimicrofilarial activity of DEC was also observed against *W. bancrofti*, *B. malayi*, *O. volvulus*, and *Loa loa* infection in humans [14–17]. DEC acts rapidly by stimulating the host immune system. In some reports macrofilaricidal effect of DEC was also recorded along with its antimicrofilarial activity [18–21]. Peixoto et al. [22] described the direct mechanism of action of this drug during their in vitro and in vivo studies; they observed apoptosis and organelle damage of *W. bancrofti* microfilariae by DEC [22]. To enhance the effect of DEC against microfilariae, nitric oxide was induced by some researchers and was found to be a good synergist [23]. However, DEC combined with albendazole [24] revealed an effective killing of *W. bancrofti* microfilariae, but the combination therapy increased the development of hydroceles in the treated patient [25].

7.2 Ivermectin (IVM)

It is a broad-spectrum anthelmintic and an effective macrofilaricidal drug introduced in 1981 also known as Mectizan [2], which was the first commercially available macrocyclic lactone. Chemically, it is a 22,23-dihydro semisynthetic derivative of avermectin B1, which is a fermentation product of actinomycetes *S. avermitilis* discovered by Merck in the mid-1970s [11–32]. IVM alone or in combination with DEC [8] resulted in long-term suppression of microfilariae in both bancroftian and brugian filariasis [20, 33, 34].

7.3 Suramin

Suramin [35] initially was a drug used to cure trypanosomiasis and onchocerciasis. Chemically it is an 8,80-(carbonylbis[imino-3,1-phenylenecarbonylimino(4-methyl-3,1-phenylene)carbonylimino])bis-1,3,5-naphthalenetrisulfonic acid hexasodium salt. Presently it is the only macrofilaricidal drug that is effective against *W. bancrofti* and *O. volvulus*.

7.4 Albendazole

This anthelmintic drug is [24] a benzimidazole derivative. Recently this has been used in a clinical trial to check out its efficacy as antifilarial drug [36]. Its efficacy was increased when administered in combination with either DEC [8] or IVM [2].

Antifilarial agent	Recommended dose	Route of administration	Mechanism of action	Filarial worm	Side effects
Diethyl carbamazine (piperazine derivative)	6 mg/kg for 12 days (individual treatment) 6 mg/kg in 24 hours (weekly/monthly/single annual dose in mass treatment) for treating *W. bancrofti* infection	Oral	Alterations in arachidonic acid metabolism of host endothelial cells and microfilariae, resulting in blood vessel constriction and host granulocyte and platelet aggregation; apoptosis and org nelle damage	*W. bancrofti* infection	Encephalitis and retinal hemorrhage. Increasing dose include systemic reaction: nausea, GIT upset, malaise, body aches, and anorexia. Localized reactions: abscess formation, lymphadenitis, and transient lymphedema
	3–5 mg/kg for 6–12 days (individual treatment) 3–5 mg/kg in 24 hours (6 times at weekly or monthly in mass treatment) for treating *B. malayi* and *B. timori* infections			*B. malayi* and *B. timori* infections	
	8 mg/kg for 14 days For the treatment of occult filariasis			Occult filariasis	
Table salt + Diethylcarbamazine	0.1% for 6 months treatment of LF			*W. bancrofti* (lymphatic filariasis)	
	0.3% for 3–4 months *B. malayi* is endemic			*B. malayi*	
Ivermectin (macrocyclic lactone)	400 mg/kg single dose treatment 4800 mg/kg for 6 months treatment *of B. malayi* and single dose remove microfilariae *W. bancrofti*	Oral	Targets glutamate gated Cl- and K+ ion channels in nematodes, results in hyperpolarization that causes paralysis of the body wall muscle and pharynx. The drug also affects ligand-gated chloride ion channels gated by GABA. It competes with retinol for the retinol-binding site on retinol-binding proteins (RBPs) in the parasite only	Bancroftian and brugian filariasis	Same as DEC, and special care must be considered, such as avoiding its use in cases of pregnancy and in children younger than 5 years old
Suramin	63.7 mg/kg in 6 incremental weekly doses (3.3, 6.7, 10.0, 13.3, 15.7, 16.7 mg/kg for the first and sixth weeks, respectively)	Intravenous (10% solution in water)	It adversely affects enzymes associated with glucose catabolism and destabilizes DNA and protein kinase enzymes in filarial worms	*W. bancrofti*, *O. volvulus*	Fatal collapse, albuminuria, ulceration, and persistent high fever; polyuria, tiredness, tenderness, anorexia, and increased thirst; among others are some of the milder side effects

Antifilarial agent	Recommended dose	Route of administration	Mechanism of action	Filarial worm	Side effects
Levimazol	An initial dose of 100 mg followed by the same dose twice daily for 10 days was found to be as effective as the total oral dosage of DEC at 126 mg per kg body weight	Oral	Acts as nicotinic receptor agonist that causes prolonged activation of the excitatory nicotinic acetylcholine (nACh) receptors on the body wall muscle of parasites, leading to spastic muscle paralysis in the worm	*W. bancrofti*, *B. malayi*	No side effects at recommended doses
Albendazole (benzimidazole) Albendazole+ DEC	Albendazole (400 mg) + diethylcarbamazine (DEC) (6 mg/kg)	Oral	Block tubulin polymerization, thereby inhibiting microtubule formation. It also inhibits parasite intestinal cells, preventing glucose uptake leading to the death of the parasite	Macrofilaricidal	Embryotoxicity and teratogenicity
Albendazole+ ivermectin	Albendazole (400 mg) + ivermectin (150–200 mg/kg)				

Table 3.
Summary of the recommended doses of currently used antifilarials.

DOI: http://dx.doi.org/10.5772/intechopen.89454

Antifilarial agent	Action	Parasite	Dose	Reference
Trisubstituted pyrimidine derivatives (the amino group and 4-aminophenyl group at the second position plays an important role in exerting antifilarial activity)	ATP-dependent DNA topoisomerase II inhibitory activity	*S. cervi*	10–40 mg/ml	[38, 39]
2-Sulfanyl-6-methyl-1,4-dihydropyrimidines		*B. malayi* (in vitro) *B. malayi–Mastomys coucha*	25 and 50 μM 100 mg/kg	
Indole derivatives B-carboline		*L. carinii–S. hispidus* (cotton rats) *A. viteae–M. natalensis*	30 mg/kg for 5 days 50 mg/kg for 5 days	[40–43]
b-Carbolines (substituted 9Hpyrido[3,4-b] indoles)		*L. carinii, A. viteae* and *B. malayi* in a *M. coucha* model	50 mg/kg for 5 days	
Quinoline and related compounds 7-chloro-4-(substituted amino)quinolines		*A. viteae*		[44–47]
3-Nitro-4-quinolones via ipso-nitration	Thymidylate kinase inhibitory activity	*Brugia malayi*	IC50 2.9 mM	
Quinolones compound 7-chloro-4-(substituted amino)quinolines	Evaluation against DNA topoisomerase II enzyme, compound	Screened in vivo against *A. viteae*	200 mg/kg for 5 days	
3-Nitro-4-quinolones	*Brugia malayi* thymidylate kinase inhibitory activity	*B. malayi*	IC50 2.9 mM	
Glycoside cinnamoyl glycosides		*S. cervi*	MIC (3.40 nM), IC50 (6.90 nM) and LC50 (25 nM) values, CC50 value of approximately 103 nM	[48]
Cinnamoyl glycosides	Chromatin condensation and DNA fragmentation; this compound also damaged the cuticular sheath of the microfilariae	*W. bancrofti*	MIC and IC50 values were 4.4 nM/ml and 8.96 nM/ml, respectively	
Dioxocine 3,6-epoxy dioxocines		*B. malayi–M. coucha*	IC50 values (0.4 mg/ml and 1.8 mg/ml, with selectivity indices (SI) of 100 and 22.2 with respect to macrofilariae and microfilariae, respectively	[49]

Antifilarial agent	Action	Parasite	Dose	Reference
Compound		*B. malayi* in jirid	Found to be potent in terms of both in vitro (IC50 1.6 mg/ml and 3.5 mg/ml for macrofilariae and microfilariae, respectively) and in vivo antifilarial activity, 200 mg/kg	
Alcohols cyclohexanol, 2- substituted propanol Cyclooctanol derivatives		*A. viteae* and *L. carinii* in rodents *A. viteae* in rodent	100% macrofilaricidal activity (at a dose of 200 mg/kg for 5 days) 81% sterilization of female worms (at a dose of 100 mg/kg for 5 days) against	[50]
Triazine	DHFR (dihydrofolate reductase) inhibitors, good inhibitory activity (approximately 74%) against PARP (polyadenosine diphosphate ribose polymerase)enzyme	*B. malayi*	Almost 100% loss of motility of filarial worms at 20 mg/ml showed better activity (IC_{50} 10.90 mM) when compared with standard antifolate (positive control) compounds, i.e., trimethoprim (IC_{50} 12.92 mM) and pyrimethamine (IC_{50} 20.10 mM	[51, 52]
Benzopyran (coumarin)		*B. malayi–M. coucha* *B. malayi*–jirid model	When administered orally at a dose of 300 mg/kg for 5 days showed 53.6% macrofilaricidal and 46% microfilaricidal activity At a dose of 100 mg/ kg for 5 days, showed 75% adulticidal and 50% microfilaricidal activity	[53–55]
Naphthalene derivative 1,4-naphthoquinones	1,3-Dimethyl substitution on the butylamino side chain favors an increased lipophilicity with potentially improved binding to the active site, which results in elevated macrofilaricidal activity (133)	*Setaria digitata*	ED50 value of 2.6 mM after a 24 h incubation and 0.91 mM after a 48 h incubation	[56]
Thiazolidine heterocyclic thiazolidine compounds compound (31) and compound (32)		*B. malayi*	IC50 values of 5.2 mM and 1.78 mM LD50 values of 349 mM and 17.59 mM, respectively	[14]

Antifilarial agent	Action	Parasite	Dose	Reference
Butylated hydroxy anisole (BHA)	Oxidative stress-induced apoptosis was found to be its major killing mechanism (135)	*S. cervi*	At 100 mM was found to be a potent adulticide	[15]
Piperazine benzoyl piperazine derivatives (two compounds, viz., compound (34) and compound (35) containing a 4-chloro (para) substituent and 3-methyl (meta) substituent on the aromatic ring)		*S. cervi*	Worms were immotile following treatment with these two compounds at a concentration of 8 mg ml 1	[16, 17, 57]
Pyrrolidine chalcone derivative (36) containing the pyrrolidine-methoxy group	Showed a significant suppression of glutathione-S-transferase (GST) activity in the macrofilariae of female *S. cervi* at a concentration of 3 mM in vitro	*S. cervi*	100% inhibition	
Diaminoalkane N1,Nn-xylofuranosylated diaminoalkanes		*B. malayi–M. coucha* *B. malayi–jirid*	At 50 mg kg 1 provided approximately 38.7% recovery of macrofilariae and 63.80% sterilization of female parasites The same compound also showed 33.5% adulticidal action along with 50% sterilization of female worms	[58]
Secondary amines		*A. viteae*	At a dose of 200 mg/kg for 5 days exhibited 100% macrofilaricidal activity, whereas compound elicited a microfilaricidal response of approximately 93%	[59]
Glycyrrhetinic acid derivatives and the benzylamide analog		*B. malayi*	Killing microfilariae and macrofilariae at 50 and 25 mM, respectively The IC50 values were found to be 2.2 mM against microfilariae and 8.8 mM against macrofilariae of the worm	[60]
		B. malayi–jirid	At a dose of 100 mg/kg for 5 days exhibited 40% adulticidal activity	

Antifilarial agent	Action	Parasite	Dose	Reference
Nitazoxanide and tizoxanide	The researchers further reported that both compounds reduced microfilarial production and impaired embryogenesis in female worms. They also suggested that mitochondria in the worms may be a possible target of NTZ (41) and TZ (42) because in addition to damaged worm tissues, they found alterations in the mitochondria	*B. malayi*	Macrofilariae were found completely immotile after 6 days when cultured with these two compounds at concentrations of 20 mg/ml On day 8 of culture at concentrations of 2.5 mg/ml, both drugs also caused a 50% decrease in worm viability Microfilarial motility was also hampered by these compounds at concentrations exceeding 5 mg/ml, and the worms were completely immotile following treatment with 20 mg/ml (after 48 h)	[61]
Nitazoxanide Nitazoxanide + silver nanoparticles	Inhibit TCA cycle enzymes	*S. cervi*	100% mortality of microfilariae at 100 µg/ml 100% mortality of microfilariae at 30 µg/ml	[62, 63]
Anthraquinone 3-methylcatechol with a substitution of acylium ions	Marked effects on intrauterine embryos of parasite	*B. malayi* infection in humans	At 5 ppm (18–19 mM) showed 100% mortality within 1, 5, and 3 days against microfilariae and adult male and female worms	[64]
Sulfonamide sulfonamide chalcones		*B. malayi*	IC50 value was found to be 4.4 mM, LD50 value of 188 mMt 500 mM concentration after 48 h of incubation	[65]
Benzothiazole novel chalcone–benzothiazole hybrids	It showed higher binding interactions at the active site of BmTMK (*B. malayi* thymidylate kinase, an essential enzyme for nucleotide metabolism in B. *malayi*).	*B. malayi*	IC50 values of 2.12 mM and 1.63 mM, respectively, for adult worms as well as microfilariae MIC value of 5 mM for both the forms IC_{50} value was 95.3 mM	[66]
Thiazole chalcone–thiazole derivatives		*B. malayi–jirid* *B. malayi–M. coucha*	At a dose of 100 mg/kg for 5 days showed 100% embryostatic activity Exerted approximately 49% macrofilaricidal activity and	[67]

Antifilarial agent	Action	Parameter	Dose	Reference
Benzimidazole derivatives HOE 33258 mebendazole, Flubendazole 2,2′-Dicarbomethoxyamino-5,5′-dibenzimidazolyl ketone	At 5 × 2.5 mg/kg and 1 × 25 mg/kg in jirds and 1 × 100 mg/kg in cats when administered by subcutaneous injection A dose of 3 mg/kg (i.p.) and 50 mg/kg (oral) × 5 days of Comp. 82/437 At a dose of 150 and 200 mg/kg for 5 days	*L. carinii* and *D. immitis* Evaluated in jirds (*Meriones unguiculatus*) and cats (*Felis catus*) infected with *Brugia pahangi* *L. carinii* in cotton rats *Dipetalonema viteae* and *Brugia malayi* in *Mastomys natalensis*	Macrofilaricidal. It also killed developing larvae in jirds. It was not microfilaricidal Eliminated almost 100% of adult worms and microfilariae It killed 100% of the macrofilariae and 97% of the microfilariae	[68–79]
Silver	Nanosilver	*B. malayi*	LD_{50} concentration (by trypan blue exclusion) of 101.2 mM and an IC_{50} value of 50.6 mM (complete microfilariae population found immotile). At 4.6 mM only, nanosilver caused a 50% decrease in the motility of the parasite	[80]

Table 4.
List of synthetic and naturally originated antifilarials.

Plant	Extract	Target	Antifilarial efficiency	Author
Streptomyces sp. 17,944	Three new tirandamycins	*B. malayi*	Inhibit the asparaginyl-tRNA-synthetase (BmAsnRS) enzyme at an IC50 value of 30 mM	[81]
Streptomyces sp. 9078	Depsipeptide	*B. malayi*	IC50 value of 50 mM	[82]
Streptomyces sp. 4875	Four adipostatins (alkyl resorcinols) potent among the compounds	*B. malayi*	Kill the worms at 1 mM concentrations	[83]
Lantana camara	Crude extract	*A. viteae*	LC_{100} 62.5 μg/ml	[84]
		B. malayi	LC_{100} 500 mg/ml	
	Chloroform, n-butanol and aqueous	*B. malayi*	LC_{100} 250 μg/ml	
	Fractions of n-hexane oleanonic acid	*B. malayi*	LC_{100} 31.25 μg/ml	
	Oleanonic acid		LC100 62.5 μg/ml	
	Crude extract 1 g/kg × 5 days	*A. viteae/M. coucha* model	95.05% reduction in Mf 23.65% effective against adult	
		B. malayi transplanted/ M. unguiculatus	80% effective against adult	
Taxodium distichum	A001 (crude ethanolic extract of aerial part) F001 (hexane fraction) K003(labda-8(20),13-diene-15-oic acid) and K004 (metasequoic acid A) SF1 (fraction) SF_4 (fraction)	*B. malayi*	mf (LC100 3.91 μg/ml) than adult worms (LC_{100} 15.63 μg/ml) IC_{50} values for the respective parasite stages were found to be 1.95 and 10.00 μg/ml mf (LC100 7.83 μg/ml) adult worms (LC100 31.25 μg/ml) mf (LC_{100} 31.25 μg/ml) and adult worms (LC_{100} 125 μg/ml) mf (LC_{100} 7.83 μg/ml) than adult (LC_{100} 31.25 μg/ml) mf (LC_{100} 62.5 μg/ml) adult (LC_{100} 125 μg/ml)	[85]
	A001 (500 mg/kg × 5 days; orally) K003 (100 mg/kg × 5 days) exerted At 100 mg/kg dose, both K003 and K004 K003 (100 mg/kg × 5 days)	*B. malayi/M. unguiculatus* *B. malayi/M. coucha model*	100% effective against Adult >95%; remarkable embryostatic activity Produced >25% macrofilaricidal activity Exerted 53.94% macrofilaricidal	

Plant	Extract	Target	Antifilarial efficiency	Author
Azadirachta indica	Alcoholic extract of flowers Aqueous extract of flowers	*S. cervi*	Mf(LC50 of 15 ng/ml) (LC90 ¼ 23 ng/ ml), mf(LC50 of 18 ng/ml) (LC90 ¼ 25 ng/ ml)	[86–88]
	Methanolic extract of leaves Ethanolic extract of leaves	*S. cervi*	Mf 100% mortality at 200 μg/ml in 135 min Mf 90% mortality at 200 μg/ml in 135 min	
	Ethanolic extract of *A. indica* leaves	*S. cervi*	Showed significant worm reduction at 25 lg/ml and highest mortality at 100 lg/ml after 24 h of incubation when applied against the microfilariae	
Eucalyptus tereticornis	Ursolic acid obtained from the leaves	*B. malayi*	LC100 50 mM and IC50 8.84 mM against microfilariae, and LC100 100 mM and IC50 35.36 mM against adult worms	[89]
Senecio nudicaulis	Aqueous leaf extract Alcoholic leaf extract	*Setaria cervi*	Both the extracts exhibited macrofilaricidal activity LC50 10 ng/ml and LC90 15 ng/ml LC50 5 ng/ml and LC90 12 ng/ml	[90]
Hibiscus sabdariffa	n-Butanol insoluble fraction of leaf extract	*B. malayi*	At 250 mg/ml concentration demonstrated a high microfilarial motility	[91]
	At a dose of 500 mg/kg × 5 days 1 g/kg × 5 days	*B. malayi*–jirid model *B. malayi*–M. *coucha* model	Showed 30% macrofilaricidal activity Showed 57% macrofilaricidal activity	
Trachyspermum ammi	Methanolic extract of fruit The 2-isopropyl-5-methyl phenol (thymol) was the active component Its positional isomer (i.e., 5-isopropyl-2-methyl phenol, carvacrol,) also showed promising result	*S. digitata*	IC_{50} 0.067 and 0.019 mg/ml after 24 h and 48 h, respectively IC_{50} were 0.024 mg/ml and 0.002 mg/ml after 24 h and 48 h incubation, respectively Macrofilaricidal IC_{50} values were 0.025 mg/ml and 0.004 mg/ml after 24 h and 48 h incubation, respectively.	[92]
	2-Isopropyl-5-methyl phenol at a dose of 50 mg/ kg for 5 days	*B. malayi–M. coucha*	Macrofilarial mortality of 58.93%	

Plant	Extract	Target	Antifilarial efficiency	Author
Bauhinia racemosa (B. racemosa)	Galactolipid (n-butanol fraction) obtained from ethanolic extraction of the leaves	*B. malayi*	The MIC values against adult worms 3.9 mg/ml and 15.6 mg/ml against microfilariae The IC_{50} values were 1.25 mg/ml and 1.607 mg/ml, respectively, against adult worms and microfilariae	[93]
	50 mg/kg × 5 days	*B. malayi infection*	58.3% adult worm mortality	
Piper betel	Crude methanolic at a dose of 100 mg/kg	*B. malayi–M. coucha*	Suppress mf most effectively and showed 26% efficacy against adult worm	[94]
Hibiscus mutabilis	Active ferulic acid, from the leaves	*S. cervi*	Approximately 97 and 90%, of reductions in viability of microfilariae and adult worms, respectively	[95]
Caesalpinia bonducella	Crude extract from the seed kernel	*B. malayi*	96% macrofilaricidal activity	[96]
Melaleuca cajuputi	The flower extract	*B. pahangi*	Halted the release of mf and worm mobility after 6 days at 1000 mg/ml	[97]
Xylocarpus granatum	Aqueous–ethanolic extract fruit extract	*B. malayi*	IC_{50} value of 15.46 and 13.17 mg/ml against macrofilariae and microfilariae, respectively	[98]
	The ethyl acetate soluble fraction demonstrated		An IC_{50} value of 8.5 and 6.9 mg ml^{-1} against macrofilariae and microfilariae, respectively	
	At a dose of 50 mg/kg for 5 days	*B. malayi–M. coucha*	53% macrofilaricidal and 63% embryostatic effects	
	Gedunin (64) Photogedunin		Mf (IC_{50} 2.03 mg/ml) Adult (IC_{50} 0.239 mg/ml) Mf (IC_{50} 2.23 mg/ml) Adult (IC_{50} 0.213 mg/ml)	
	Gedunin at a dose of 100 mg/kg for 5 days Photogedunin at a dose of 100 mg/kg for 5 days	*B. malayi–M. coucha*	Killed 80.0% of the transplanted adult worms 70.0% adult worm mortality	
Vitex negundo (V. negundo) and *Aegle marmelos (A. marmelos)*	The root extract *from V. negundo* and the leaf extract from *A. marmelos*	*B. malayi*	At a concentration of 100 ng/ml caused a complete loss of microfilarial motility after 48 h of incubation	[99]
Aegle marmelos	Methanolic extracts of *Aegle marmelos* Corr. (Rutaceae) leaves	*S. cervi*	(IC_{50}) was 0.168 mg/ml	[100]

DOI: http://dx.doi.org/10.5772/intechopen.89454

Plant	Extract	Target	Antifilarial efficiency	Author
Diospyros peregrina	n-Butanol extract (NBE) of *D. peregrina* stem bark on *Setaria cervi*	*S. cervi*	Mf (IC_{50} 56.1 μg/ml, (IC_{50}), adult (IC_{50} 57.6 μg/ml) Mf (LD100 187.17 μg/ml) after 24 h of treatment	[101]
Cajanus scarabaeoides (L)	The polyphenol-rich ethanolic extract obtained from the stem part	*S. cervi*	LD_{50} values were 2.5, 10 and 35 μg/ml, against the oocytes, microfilariae (Mf) and adults, respectively	[102]
Ficus racemosa	Alcoholic and aqueous extract of fruits of *F. racemosa*	*Setaria cervi*	LC_{50} and LC_{90} were 21 and 35 ng/ml, respectively, for alcoholic, while for aqueous extracts were 27 and 42 ng/ml, respectively	[103]
Botryocladia leptopoda	The crude ethanolic extract from the marine red alga *B. leptopoda*	*A. viteae* *L. sigmodontis* *Brugia malayi*	LC_{100} of 62.5 mg ml^{-1} LC_{100} of 31.25 mg ml^{-1} LC_{100} of 125 mg ml^{-1}	[104]
	At a dose of 200 mg/kg for 5 days	*L. sigmodontis–cotton rats* *A. viteae–M. coucha and* *B. malayi–M. coucha*	Exhibited 71.6% 63.2% (ethanolic extract) and 45% (hexane fraction) macrofilaricidal activity, respectively	
Haliclona oculata	The methanolic extract Chloroform fraction and its one chromatographic fraction	*B. malayi*	Mf (IC_{50} 5 mg/ml) Adult (1.88 mg/ml) Showed antimacrofilarial activity IC_{50} 1.80 mg/ml and 1.62 mg/ml, respectively, whereas concentrations of 1.72 mg/ml and 1.19 mg/ml were effective against microfilariae	[105]
	At a dose of 100 mg/kg for 5 days the methanol extract, chloroform fraction, and chromatographic fraction (contain four major alkaloids: xestospongin-C, araguspongin-C, mimosamycin, and xestospongin-D), respectively	*B. malayi–jirid*	Revealed 51.3%, 64% and 70.7% macrofilaricidal activities in the methanol extract, chloroform fraction, and chromatographic fraction, respectively.	
Haliclona exigua	Methanol extract, the n-butanol-soluble fraction Chloroform fraction Araguspongin C	*B. malayi*	(LC_{100} 31.25 mg/ml) (LC_{100} 15.6 mg/ml) Macrofilaricidal activity at 15.6 mg/ml	[106]

Plant	Extract	Target	Antifilarial efficiency	Author
Eucalyptus globulus	The leaf extract from *E. globulus* was active in vitro	*B. malayi*	IC_{50} values 62.5 and 31.2 mg/ml, respectively, against adult worms and microfilariae	[107]
	At a dose of 100 mg/kg for 5 days	*B. malayi–M. coucha model and transplanted B. malayi jirid*	Exhibited 66.7% adulticidal activity and an embryostatic effect	
Terminalia bellerica, Terminalia chebula, Terminalia catappa	Leaf extracts in different solvents	*Setaria cervi*	The methanol extract exhibited more than 80% activity at the highest dose level of 10 mg/ml. The IC_{50} obtained in methanol extracts are 2.7, 1.96 and 2.58 mg/ml	[108]
Moringa oleifera	The gum extract obtained from *M. oleifera* showed at a dose of 500 mg/kg for 5 days In contrast, at a dose of 1000 mg/kg for 5 days	*B. malayi* *B. malayi–jirid* *B. malayi–M. coucha*	Mf (LC_{100} 1000 mg/ml) Adult (LC_{100} 125 mg/ml) Mf (IC_{50} > 1000 mg/ml) Adult (IC_{50} 74.33 mg/ml) Extract showed 69% adulticidal activity and sterilized 83% of the female worms Extract showed 44% adulticidal activity	[109]
Butea monosperma	The leaf and root extract Methanol and hexane–ethanol fraction of the leaf extract	*B. malayi* *S. cervi*	Microfilarial motility in a dose-dependent manner Showed IC_{50} values of 1.25 and 3.6 mg/ml, respectively, against macrofilariae	[110, 111]
Ricinus communis	Methanolic extract of the seed	*B. malayi*	90% death in the developmental stages of the parasite	[112–114]
Rutin and hesperetin		*S. digitata*	Showed macrofilaricidal activity a 500 mg/ml	
Naringenin		*B. malayi*	Showed macrofilaricidal activity at 125 mg/ml IC_{50} value at2.5 mg/ml	
	At 50 mg/kg	*B malayi–Meriones and B. malayi-M. coucha*	Eliminate adult worms 73 and 31%, respectively	
Flavone Chrysin			Exhibit macrofilaricidal activity at 62.5 mg/ml and inhibit the adult motility at 31.2 mg/ml Showed macrofilaricidal activity at 2.50 mg/ml	

Table 5.
List of naturally originated antifilarials are summarized below.

7.5 Levamisole

This is an ascaricidal drug with no side effects at the recommended doses. It has also been found as a microfilaricidal drug against the microfilariae of *Wuchereria bancrofti* and *Brugia malayi* [37].

Unfortunately, most of the chemical antifilarials are characterized by adverse side effects. The list of currently used antifilarials with their side effects is summarized in **Table 3**. Hence, researches on exploring new therapeutic drugs, especially less hazardous drugs of natural origin, are highly recommended. The application of biomedicines to treat disease is among the oldest forms of therapy. These biomedicines including plant extracts and their secondary metabolites were believed to exert their bioefficacy through immunomodulatory elicitation of Th1/Th2 response, either by single (Th1, Th2) or mixed adjuvant activity. Therefore, in the context of filariasis, synthetic and naturally originated antifilarials are summarized in **Tables 4** and **5**.

8. Role of bioinformatics in filarial research

Bioinformatics is a science of computer-based analysis for the biological datasets in which biology and computer science are mutually helping and influencing each other in the field. Bioinformatics has increased the understanding of molecular mechanism of various cellular processes. Nowadays bioinformatics covers several fields of biological sciences and drug discovery to overcome biological problems.

8.1 Genomic approach in filarial research

Genomic research in bioinformatics is a useful technique used to understand the structure and function of all the genes within an organism. Genomics help to find the particular gene and other biological aspects in the entire genome sequence of the organism. Screening of drug targets can also be done using the genomics approach. Casiraghi et al. [115] had carried out phylogenetic analysis using bioinformatics of 11 filarial and Spirurida nematodes and identified the sequence of mitochondrial cytochrome oxidase-I (COI).

Hoerauf et al. [116] detected the mutual interaction between the intracellular bacteria (endobacteria) and filarial nematodes, which is further used as antifilarial drug targets. Nuchprayoon et al. [117] identified the genetic diversity using phylogenetic analysis parsimony tool (PAUP) between the DNA sequences of two strains of *Wb* found in Myanmar and Thailand. Ghedin et al. [118] reported the nuclear genome draft of *Bm* (95-Mb), which contains 88,363,057 bp sequences with 17.84% protein coding sequence [118]. The full genome sequences are available at NEMBASE4 database. Investigators identified a variety of filarial parasite genes and their novel functions that are involved in miRNA regulation and processing.

8.2 Proteomic approach in filarial research

Proteomics approach involved highly efficient methods of protein separation like two-dimensional-poly acrylamide gel electrophoresis (2DPAGE) and detection, using modern tools of bioinformatics. Proteomic analysis of the several stages of *Bm* has identified 557 *Bm* proteins and 11,508 protein coding genes which helps to define various proteins by using reverse-phase liquid chromatography-tandem mass spectroscopy.

Afterwards Bennuru et al. [119] have also done the same in identifying the excretory/secretory (ES) and somatic proteins of adult, mf, and infective stages of larvae of *Brugia malayi*. Some workers gathered the molecular information of the particular protein of interest through 3D structure which plays a significant role in drug designing and vaccine development for lymphatic filariasis. In 2005 Bhargavi et al. [120] analyzed the 3D model of GST of *Wuchereria bancrofti* and *Brugia malayi* for better drug development. For the development of potential drugs, novel drug targets are modeled using bioinformatics approach including either ligand-based drug designing (LBDD) or structure-based drug designing (SBDD). LBDD provides crucial understanding of the interaction between the drug target and ligand molecule and provides information about the biologically active molecules [121]. Currently 3D quantitative structural activity relationship (QSAR) and pharmacophore modeling of small molecules are carried out to define their minimum necessary structural characteristics through which it inhibits the target. These 3D structure analyses of a protein were designed from the experimental-based method such as X-ray crystallography, NMR, electron microscopy, etc. If an experimental data are not available for the target proteins, homology modeling is carried out to build the 3D structure using target protein sequence [122].

Potential inhibitor can be designed on the basis of their binding sites or can be identified from the small-sized molecule databases such as Cambridge Structural Database [123], ChemBank [124], DrugBank [125], PubChem [126], and ZINC database [127] and databases that are available at Lignad.Info: molecule database [128] to inspect the biological activity of the particular protein.

Name	Description	URL
DBEMFDD diseases database	It is an annotated bibliography for filariasis, malaria, dengue, and diarrhea. It also contains the findings of the literature survey	http://ideas.repec.org/p/ess/wpaper/id2032.html
FilaDB	Database on filaria detection, clinico-immuno monitoring, and management has been developed for Kasturba Hospital and private practitioners to screen the filarial infection	http://www.jbtdrc.org/FilaDb.htm
NEMBASE2	Contains the EST sequence for *Brugia malayi* and other nematodes	http://www.nematodes.org/nematodeESTs/nembase.html
Filaria Journal	Full and freely access journal of filariasis	*http://www.filariajournal.com/*
Wormbase	It is an online database for the biology and genome of the *Ce* and related nematodes	http://www.wormbase.org
WHO	It contains the related publication of filariasis, reports of elimination program, control of neglected tropical diseases and some important links	*http://www.who.int/topics/filariasis/en/*
PHIS	It contains the news and updated from filariasis elimination program	http://umis.doh.gov.ph/fila
Disease database	It contains the general information regarding diseases	*http://www.diseasesdatabase.com/ddb4824.htm*
TDR-lymphatic filariasis	It contains knowledge about the parasite genomes for African lymphatic filariasis and other diseases TDR is now focusing on providing capacity to use the parasite genome data and on supporting developments in applied genomics and bioinformatics	*http://www.who.int/tdrold/diseases/lymphfil/default.htm*
Filarial worms database	This database provides the genome sequence of organisms rapidly and broadly available to the scientific community.	*http://www.broadinstitute.org/annotation/genome/filarial_worms/MultiHome.html*

Table 6.
List of online databases for lymphatic filariasis are as follows.

8.3 Web-based available resources for LF

Web-based biological data plays a significant role in bioinformatics which plays a significant role in analyzing biological data for large amount of nucleotide sequences, amino acid sequences, and 2D or 3D structures for the broad range of organisms and their drug targets. Currently, there are only few databases available for LF (**Table 6**), but the specified database for LF is not available, which is an urgent need in the field of drug development and to overcome the emerging drug resistance. Some of the important databases which are available for LF research have been discussed below.

NEMBASE: It contains databases containing information of filarial nematodes such as filarial biology and pathology, nomenclature of filarial genome, mapping of filarial gene, and *Bm* genome survey sequencing (GSS). Recently, genome sequencing of *wBm* and *Onchocerca volvulus* (*Ov*) was also included with the Sanger Institute, NEB, and TIGR.

WormBase: It's an open access database repository for nematode biology which contains the genome browser for *Bm*, *C. elegans*, *H. contortus*, etc., and the gene predictions and orthology assignments from a range of related nematodes.

FilaDB: It is a database for screening filarial patients with the objective of providing information on the incidence of mf and types of acute, chronic, and occult manifestations and age, sex, and distribution area of filariasis cases for clinico-immuno monitoring and management of filariasis.

Filarial worm database at broad institute: This database used to study the minute phenotypic difference between the closely related filarial species of *Loa loa*, *Wb*, and *Ov* (*http://www.filariasiscenter.org/brugia-malayigenomics-and-bioinformatics-resources*). Filarial worm database also has the sequence data on *Wolbachia* endosymbionts of *Wb*, *Ov*, and *Bm*. Filarial diseases are still remaining as a major public health concern in India. There is a need of comprehensive database, which should contain:

a. Curated links between genes relevant to filariasis and their sequences in GenBank and Swiss-Prot.

b. Sequence homology between different filariasis causing genes.

c. Primary and secondary information of pathogens.

d. Availability of various drugs and their targets.

e. Expressed sequence tagged (EST) sequences from different filarial species.

f. Supporting references from published literatures.

g. Bioinformatics tools to analyze those data. Database should also contain the epidemiological data on age and gender-wise incidences of disease, remission, and transition rates of disease sequelae.

9. Conclusions

Filariasis is one of the most disabling and disfiguring neglected tropical diseases with various clinical manifestations and a high morbidity rate. Repetitive use of antifilarials has given rise to drug resistance. Most of them are effective against microfilariae and have no effect on the adult worms. Till date numbers of antifilarial targets have been explored, but their evaluation with reference to assay feasibility, target validation, drugability, toxicity, resistance potential, and structural information needs to be discovered in the future. There is a need to explore the mechanism through which drug resistance occurs so that new effective combination therapy could be discovered at an early stage.

Author details

Sharba Kausar
Department of Microbiology, Jawaharlal Nehru Medical College, Aligarh Muslim University, Aligarh, UP, India

*Address all correspondence to: sharbakausar@gmail.com

References

[1] World Health Organization. Global programme to eliminate lymphatic filariasis. In: Lymphatic Filariasis, Progress Report 2000–2009 and Strategic Plan 2010–2020; Geneva. 2010. pp. 1-78

[2] World Health Organization. Three more countries eliminate lymphatic filariasis. 2018. Available from: https://www.who.int/westernpacific/news/detail/08-10-2018-three-more-countries-eliminate-lymphatic-filariasis

[3] World Health Organization. Global Programme to eliminate lymphatic filariasis: Progress report, 2013. Weekly Epidemiological Record. 2014;**89**:409-418

[4] Ramaiah KD, Das PK, Michael E, Guyatt H. The economic burden of lymphatic filariasis in India. Parasitology Today. 2000;**16**(6):251-253

[5] Ton TG, Mackenzie C, Molyneux DH. The burden of mental health in lymphatic filariasis. Infectious Diseases of Poverty. 2015;**4**:1-8

[6] Meyrowitsch DW, Simonsen PE, Magesa SM. A 26-year follow-up of bancroftian filariasis in two communities in north-eastern Tanzania. Annals of Tropical Medicine and Parasitology. 2004;**98**:155-169

[7] Molyneux DH, Zagaria N. Lymphatic filariasis elimination: Progress in global programme development. Annals of Tropical Medicine and Parasitology. 2002;**96**:S15-S40

[8] World Health Organization. Sustaining the drive to overcome the global impact of neglected tropical diseases. In: Second WHO Report on Neglected Tropical Diseases, Geneva. 2013. pp. 1-137

[9] Third WHO Report on Neglected Tropical Diseases, Investing to Overcome the Global Impact of Neglected Tropical Diseases. Geneva: WHO; 2015

[10] Liu LX, Weller PF. Antiparasitic drugs. The New England Journal of Medicine. 1996;**334**:1178-1184

[11] Pink R, Hudson A, Mouriès MA, Bendig M. Opportunities and challenges in antiparasitic drug discovery. Nature Reviews Drug Discovery. 2005;**4**(9):727-740

[12] Hewitt RI, Kushner S, Stewart H, White E, Wallace W, Subbarow Y. Experimental chemotherapy of filariasis. III. Effect of 1-diethyl-carbamyl-4-methylpiperazine hydrochloride against naturally acquired filarial infections in cotton rats and dogs. Journal of Laboratory and Clinical Medicine. 1947;**32**:1314-1329

[13] Babu S, Nutman TB. Immunology of lymphatic filariasis. Parasite Immunology. 2014;**36**(8):338-346

[14] Mandvikar A, Hande SV, Yeole P, Goswami K, Reddy MVR. Therapeutic potential of novel heterocyclic thiazolidine compounds against human lymphatic filarial parasite: An *in vitro* study. International Journal of Pharmaceutical Sciences and Research. 2016;**7**(4):1480-1492

[15] Rathaur S, Yadav M, Singh N, Singh A. Effect of diethylcarbamazine, butylated hydroxy anisole and methyl substituted chalcone on filarial parasite *Setaria cervi*: proteomic and biochemical approaches. Journal of Proteomics. 2011;**74**(9):1595-1606

[16] Saxena R, Sharma S, Iyer RN, Anand N. Potential filaricides. 5.3-Ethyl-8-methyl-1,3,8-triazabicyclo[4.4.0]decan-2-one, a new antifilarial agent. Journal of Medicinal Chemistry. 1971;**14**(10):929-931

[17] Kalyanasundaram M, Mathew N, Paily KP, Prabhakaran G. Synthesis and screening of 1-methyl-4-substituted benzoyl piperazides against adult *Setaria digitata* for antifilarial activity. Acta Tropica. 2009;**111**(2):168-171

[18] Melrose W. Lymphatic Filariasis: A Review 1862–2002. Australia: Warwick Educational Publishing Inc.; 2004. pp. 1-80

[19] Weil GJ, Lammie PJ, Richards FO, Eberhard ML. Changes in circulating parasite antigen levels after treatment of bancroftian filariasis with diethylcarbamazine and ivermectin. Journal of Infectious Diseases. 1991; **164**(4):814-816

[20] Ismail MM, Weil GJ, Jayasinghe KSA, Premaratne UN, Abeyewickreme W, Rajaratnam HN, et al. Prolonged clearance of microfilaraemia in patients with Bancroftian filariasis after multiple high doses of ivermectin of diethylcarbamazine. Transactions of the Royal Society of Tropical Medicine and Hygiene. 1996;**90**:684-688

[21] McCarthy JS, Guinea A, Weil GJ, Ottesen EA. Clearance of circulating filarial antigen as a measure of the macrofilaricidal activity of diethylcarbamazine in *Wuchereria bancrofti* infection. The Journal of Infectious Diseases. 1995;**172**(2):521-526

[22] Peixoto CA, Rocha A, Aguiar-Santos A, Florencio MS. The effects of diethylcarbamazine on the ultrastructure of microfilariae of *Wuchereria bancrofti in vivo* and *in vitro*. Parasitolology Research. 2004;**92**(6): 513-517

[23] Subramanian S, Vanamail P, Das PK, Pani SP, Ravi R. Randomized controlled clinical trials of antifilarial drugs for lymphatic filariasis: Endpoints of outcome measures influence drug efficacy. In: Presented at: Proceedings of the 23rd Conference of the Indian Society for Medical Statistics, Jawaharlal Nehru Medical College, Belgaum, India, January. 2005. pp. 19-21

[24] Singh PK, Ajay A, Kushwaha S, Tripathi RP, Misra-Bhattacharya S. Towards novel antifilarial drugs: Challenges and recent developments. Future Medical Chemistry. 2010;**2**(2): 251-283

[25] Hussein O, Setouhy ME, Ahmed ES, Kandil AM, Ramzy RM, Helmy H, et al. Duplex Doppler sonographic assessment of the effects of diethylcarbamazine and albendazole therapy on adult filarial worms and adjacent host tissues in Bancroftian filariasis. American Journal of Tropical Medicine and Hygiene. 2004;**71**:471-477

[26] Mak JW. Antifilarial compounds in the treatment and control of lymphatic filariasis. Tropical Biomedicine. 2004; **21**(2):27-38

[27] Woodruff HB, Burg RW. The Antibiotics Explosion. Discoveries in Pharmacology. In: Parnhamand MJ, Bruinvels J, editors. Pharmacological Methods, Receptors and Chemotherapy. Vol. 3. Amsterdam, The Netherlands: Elsevier; 1986. pp. 338-341

[28] Thylefors B. Eliminating onchocerciasis as a public health problem. Tropical Medicine and International Health. 2004;**9**(4):A1-A3

[29] Schares G, Hofmann B, Zahner H. Antifilarial activity of macrocyclic lactones: Comparative studies with ivermectin, doramectin, milbemycin A4 oxime, and moxidectin in *Litomosoides carinii*, *Acanthocheilonema viteae*, *Brugia malayi*, and *B. pahangi* infection of *Mastomys coucha*. Tropical Medicine and Parasitology. 1994;**45**(2):97-106

[30] Campbell WC. Ivermectin as an antiparasitic agent for use in humans.

Annual Review of Microbiology. 1991; **45**:445-474

[31] Ottesen EA, Campbell WCJ. Ivermectin in human medicine. Journal of Antimicrobial Chemotherapy. 1994; **34**:195-203

[32] Townson S, Tagboto SK, Castro J, Lujan A, Awadzi K, Titanji VPK. Comparison of the sensitivity of different geographical races of *Onchocerca volvulus* microfilariae to ivermectin: Studies *in vitro*. Transactions of the Royal Society of Tropical Medicine and Hygiene. 1994; **88**:101-106

[33] Dreyer G, Noroes J, Amaral F, Nen A, Medeiros Z, Coutinho A, et al. Comparison of the sensitivity of different geographical races of *Onchocerca volvulus* microfilariae to ivermectin: Studies *in-vitro*. Transactions of the Royal Society of Tropical Medicine and Hygiene. 1995; **89**:441-443

[34] Shenoy RK, Kumaraswami V, Rajan K, Thankom S, Jalajakumari A. A comparative study of the efficacy and tolerability of single and split doses of ivermectin and diethylcarbamazine in periodic Brugian filariasis. Annals of Tropical Medicine and Parasites. 1993; **87**:459-467

[35] Simonsen PE, Malecela MN, Michael E, Mackenzie CD, editors. Lymphatic Filariasis, Research and Control in Eastern and Southern Africa. Denmark: DBL-Center for Health and Research Development; 2008. pp. 1-155

[36] McCarthy J. Is anthelmintic resistance a threat to the program to eliminate lymphatic filariasis? American Journal of Tropical Medicine and Hygiene. 2005;**73**(2):232-233

[37] Miller MJ. Use of levamisole in parasitic infections. Drugs. 1980;**20**(2): 122-130

[38] Katiyar SB, Bansal I, Saxena JK, Chauhan PMS. Syntheses of 2,4,6-trisubstituted pyrimidine derivatives as a new class of antifilarial topoisomerase II inhibitors. Bioorganic & Medicinal Chemistry Letters. 2005;**15**(1):47-50

[39] Singh BK, Mishra M, Saxena N, Yadav GP, Maulik PR, Sahoo MK, et al. Synthesis of 2-sulfanyl-6-methyl-1,4-dihydropyrimidines as a new class of antifilarial agents. European Journal of Medicinal Chemistry. 2008;**43**(12): 2717-2723

[40] Agarwal A, Agarwal SK, Singh SN, Fatma N, Chatterjee RK. *In vivo* potent antifilarial β-carbolines. Bioorganic & Medicinal Chemistry Letters. 1996;**6**(3): 225-228

[41] Srivastava SK, Agarwal A, Chauhan PMS, Agarwal SK, Bhaduri AP, Singh SN, et al. Potent 1,3-disubstituted-9H-pyrido[3,4-b] indoles as new lead compounds in antifilarial chemotherapy. Journal of Medicinal Chemistry. 1999;**42**(9):1667-1672

[42] Hewitt RI, Kushner S, Stewart H, White E, Wallace WS, Subbarow Y. Experimental chemotherapy of filariasis. III. Effect of 1-diethylcarbamyl-4-methylpiperazine hydrochloride against naturally acquired filarial infections in cotton rats and dogs. Journal of Laboratory and Clinical Medicine. 1947;**32**(11): 1314-1329

[43] World Health Organization. Report of the Seventh Meeting of the Scientific Working Group on Filariasis: Filaricide Screeners TDR/Fil/SWG(7)82,3. Geneva: World Health Organization; 1982

[44] Tewari S, Chauhan PMS, Bhaduri AP, Fatima N, Chatterjee RK. Syntheses and antifilarial profile of 7-chloro-4-(substituted amino) quinolines: A new class of antifilarial agents. Bioorganic & Medicinal

Chemistry Letters. 2000;**10**(13): 1409-1412

[45] Azad SC, Balaramnavar VM, Khan IA, Doharey PK, Saxena JK, Saxena AK. Operative conversions of 3-carboxy-4-quinolones into 3-nitro-4-quinolones *via ipso*-nitration: Potential antifilarial agents as inhibitors of *Brugia malayi* thymidylate kinase. RSC Advances. 2015;**5**(100):82208-82214

[46] Srivastava SK, Chauhan PMS, Agarwal SK, Bhaduri AP, Singh SN, Fatima N, et al. Syntheses and antifilarial profile of 5-amino and 5,8-diamino-isoquinoline derivatives: A new class of antifilarial agents. Bioorganic & Medicinal Chemistry Letters. 1996;**6**(22):2623-2628

[47] Srivastava SK, Chauhan PMS, Bhaduri AP, Fatima N, Chatterjee AK. Quinolones: Novel probes in antifilarial chemotheraphy. Journal of Medicinal Chemistry. 2000;**43**(11):2275-2279

[48] Roy P, Dhara D, Parida PK, Kar RJ, Bhunia A, Jana K, et al. *C*-cinnamoyl glycosides as a new class of anti-filarial agents. European Journal of Medicinal Chemistry. 2016;**114**:308-317

[49] Sashidhara KV, Kumar A, Rao KB, Kushwaha V, Saxena K, Murthy PK. *In vitro* and *in vivo* antifilarial activity evaluation of 3,6-epoxy [1,5] dioxocines: A new class of antifilarial agents. Bioorganic & Medicinal Chemistry Letters. 2012;**22**(4):1527-1532

[50] Agarwal A, Awasthi SK, Murthy PK. *In vivo* antifilarial activity of some cyclic and acylic alcohols. Medicinal Chemistry Research. 2011;**20**(4): 430-434

[51] Sharma RD, Bag S, Tawari NR, Degani MS, Goswami K, Reddy MVR. Exploration of 2,4-diaminopyrimidine and 2,4-diamino-s-triazine derivatives as potential antifilarial agents. Parasitology. 2013;**140**(8):959-965

[52] Bag S, Tawari NR, Sharma R, Goswami K, Reddy MV, Degani MS. *In vitro* biological evaluation of biguanides and dihydrotriazines against *Brugia malayi* and folate reversal studies. Acta Tropica. 2010;**113**(1):48-51

[53] Tripathi RP, Tripathi R, Bhaduri AP, Singh SN, Chatterjee RK, Murthy PK. Antifilarial activity of some 2H-1-benzopyran-2-ones (coumarins). Acta Tropica. 2000;**76**(2):101-106

[54] Tripathi RP, Tiwari VK, Misra-Bhattacharya S, Tyagi K, Srivastava VML, Murthy PK. 7-O-[4-methyl piperazine-1-(2-acetyl)]-2H-1-benzopyran-2-one: A novel antifilarial lead compound. Acta Tropica. 2003; **87**(2):215-224

[55] Misra S, Singh LK, Gupta PJ, Misra-Bhattacharya S, Katiyar D. Synthesis and biological evaluation of 4-oxycoumarin derivatives as a new class of antifilarial agents. European Journal of Medicinal Chemistry. 2015;**94**:211-217

[56] Mathew N, Karunan T, Srinivasan L, Muthuswamy K. Synthesis and screening of substituted 1,4-naphthoquinones (NPQs) as antifilarial agents. Drug Development Research. 2010;**71**:188-196

[57] Awasthi SK, Mishra N, Dixit SK, Singh A, Yadav M, Yadav SS, et al. Antifilarial activity of 1,3-diarylpropen-1-one: Effect on glutathione-S-transferase, a phase II detoxification enzyme. American Journal of Tropical Medicine and Hygiene. 2009;**80**(5): 764-768

[58] Tiwari VK, Tewari N, Katiyar D, Tripathi RP, Arora K, Gupta S, et al. Synthesis and antifilarial evaluation of N1,Nn-xylofuranosylated diaminoalkanes. Bioorganic & Medicinal Chemistry. 2003;**11**(8):1789-1800

[59] Srivastava SK, Chauhan PMS, Bhaduri AP, Murthy PK, Chatterjee RK.

Secondary amines as new pharmacophores for macrofilaricidal drug design. Bioorganic & Medicinal Chemistry Letters. 2000;**10**(4):313-314

[60] Kalani K, Kushwaha V, Verma R, Murthy KP, Srivastava SK. Glycyrrhetinic acid and its analogs: A new class of antifilarial agents. Bioorganic & Medicinal Chemistry Letters. 2013;**23**(9):2566-2570

[61] Rao RU, Huang Y, Fischer K, Fischer PU, Weil GJ. *Brugia malayi*: Effects of nitazoxanide and tizoxanide on adult worms and microfilariae of filarial nematodes. Experimental Parasitology. 2008;**121**(1):38-45

[62] Kausar S, Khan W, Azam A. The effect of DEC, NTZ and NTZ + AgNPs on the TCA cycle enzymes of the microfilariae of *Setaria cervi in vitro*. Asian Journal of Pharmacy and Pharmacology. 2016;**2**(6):154-161

[63] Kausar S, Khan W. Comparative efficacy of diethylcarbamazine, nitazoxanide and nanocomposite of nitazoxanide and silver nanoparticles on the dehydrogenases of TCA cycle in *Setaria cervi, in vitro*. Iranian Journal of Parasitology. 2018;**13**(3):399-405

[64] Dhananjeyan MR, Milev YP, Kron MA, Nair MG. Synthesis and activity of substituted anthraquinones against a human filarial parasite, *Brugia malayi*. Journal of Medicinal Chemistry. 2005;**48**(8):2822-2830

[65] Bahekar SP, Hande SV, Agarwal NR, Chandak HS, Bhoj PS, Goswami K, et al. Sulfonamide chalcones: Synthesis and *in vitro* exploration for therapeutic potential against *Brugia malayi*. European Journal Medicinal Chemistry. 2016;**124**:262-269

[66] Sashidhara KV, Avula SR, Doharey PK, Singh LR, Balaramnavar VM, Gupta J, et al. Designing, synthesis of selective and high-affinity chalcone-benzothiazole hybrids as *Brugia malayi* thymidylate kinase inhibitors: *In vitro* validation and docking studies. European Journal Medicinal Chemistry. 2015;**103**:418-428

[67] Sashidhara KV, Rao KB, Kushwaha V, Modukuri RK, Verma R, Murthy PK. Synthesis and antifilarial activity of chalcone–thiazole derivatives against a human lymphatic filarial parasite, *Brugia malayi*. European Journal of Medicinal Chemistry. 2014; **81**:473-480

[68] Raether W, Lammler G. The filaricidal effect of basically substituted 2,6-bis-benzimidazoles in *Litomosoides carinii* infection of the cotton rat (*Sigmodon hispidus*). Annals of Tropical Medicine and Parasitology. 1971;**65**(1): 107-115

[69] Denham DA, Suswillo RR, Rogers R. The anthelmintic effects of flubendazole on *Brugia pahangi*. Transactions of the Royal Society of Tropical Medicine and Hygiene. 1978;**72**:546-547

[70] Denham DA, Samad R, Cho SY, Suswillo RR, Skippins SC. The anthelmintic effects of flubendazole on *Brugia pahangi*. Transactions of the Royal Society of Tropical Medicine and Hygiene. 1979;**73**:673-676

[71] Dominguez-Vazquez A, Taylor HR, Ruvalcaba-Macias AM, Murphy RP, Greene BM, Rivas-Alcala AR, et al. Comparison of flubendazole and diethylcarbamazine in treatment of onchocerciasis. Lancet. 1983;**1**:139-143

[72] Denham DA. Anthelmintic properties of flubendazole against *Dipetalonema viteae* in jirds. Transactions of the Royal Society of Tropical Medicine and Hygiene. 1980; **74**(6):829

[73] Reddy AB, Rao UR, Chandrashekar R, Shrivastava R, Subrahmanyam D. Comparative

efficacy of some benzimidazoles and amoscanate (Go.9333) against experimental filarial infections. Tropenmedizin und Parasitologie. 1983; **34**(4):259-262

[74] Maertens K, Wery M. Effect of mebendazole and levamisole on *Onchocerca volvulus* and *Dipetalonema perstans*. Transactions of the Royal Society of Tropical Medicine and Hygiene. 1975;**69**:359-360

[75] World Health Organization. Technical Report Series 702. In: Lymphatic Filariasis. 1984

[76] Fatima N, Sharma S, Chatterjee RK. 2,2′-Dicarbomethoxyamino-5,5′-dibenzimidazolyl ketone—A new antifilarial agent. Acta Tropica. 1989;**46**: 311-321

[77] Ram S, Wise DS, Wotring LL, McCall JW, Townsend LB. Synthesis and biological activity of certain alkyl 5-(alkoxycarbonyl)-1H-benzimidazole-2-carbamates and related derivatives: A new class of potential antineoplastic and antifilarial agents. Journal of Medicinal Chemistry. 1992;**35**(3):539-547

[78] O'Neill M, Mansour A, DiCosty U, Geary J, Dzimianski M, McCall SD, et al. An *in vitro/in vivo* model to analyze the effects of flubendazole exposure on adult female *Brugia malayi*. PLoS Neglected Tropical Diseases. 2016; **10**(5):e0004698

[79] O'Neill M, Ballesteros C, Tritten L, Burkman E, Zaky WI, Xia J, et al. Profiling the macrofilaricidal effects of flubendazole on adult female *Brugia malayi* using RNAseq. International Journal of Parasitology: Drugs and Drug Resistance. 2016;**6**(3):288-296

[80] Singh SK, Goswami K, Sharma RD, Reddy MVR, Dash D. Novel microfilaricidal activity of nanosilver. International Journal of Nanomedicine. 2012;**7**:1023-1030

[81] Yu Z, Vodanovic-Jankovic S, Ledeboer N, Huang SX, Rajski SR, Kron M, et al. Tirandamycins from *Streptomyces* sp. 17944 inhibiting the parasite *Brugia malayi* asparagine tRNA synthetase. Organic Letters. 2011;**13**(8):2034-2037

[82] Yu Z, Vodanovic-Jankovic S, Kron M, Shen B. New WS9326A congeners from *Streptomyces* sp. 9078 inhibiting *Brugia malayi* asparaginyl-tRNA synthetase. Organic Letters. 2012; **14**(18):4946-4949

[83] Rateb ME, Yang D, Vodanovic-Jankovic S, Yu Z, Kron MA, Shen B. Adipostatins A–D from *Streptomyces* sp. 4875 inhibiting *Brugia malayi* asparaginyl-tRNA synthetase and killing adult *Brugia malayi* parasites. The Journal of Antibiotics. 2015;**68**:540-542

[84] Misra N, Sharma M, Raj K, Dangi A, Srivastava S, Misra-Bhattacharya S. Chemical constituents and antifilarial activity of *Lantana camara* against human lymphatic filariid *Brugia malayi* and rodent filariid *Acanthocheilonema viteae* maintained in rodent hosts. Parasitology Research. 2007;**100**(3): 439-448

[85] Kushwaha V, Saxena K, Verma R, Katoch D, Kumar N, Lal B, et al. Antifilarial activity of diterpenoids from *Taxodium distichum*. Parasites Vectors. 2016;**9**(1):132

[86] Mishra V, Parveen N, Singhal KC, Khan NU. Antifilarial activity of *Azadirachta indica* on cattle filarial parasite *Setaria cervi*. Fitoterapia. 2005; **76**(1):54-61

[87] Mukherjee N, Saini P, Mukherjee S, Roy P, Babu SPS. *In vitro* antifilarial activity of *Azadirachta indica* aqueous extract through reactive oxygen species enhancement. Asian Pacific Journal of Tropical Medicine. 2014;**7**(11):841-848

[88] Kausar S. *In vitro* evaluation of antifilarial effect of *Azadirachta indica*

leaves extract in different solvents on the microfilariae of *Setaria cervi*. Journal of Parasitic Diseases. 2016;**41**(1):9-15

[89] Kalani K, Kushwaha V, Sharma P, Verma R, Srivastava M, Khan F, et al. *In vitro, in silico* and *in vivo* studies of ursolic acid as an anti-filarial agent. PLoS One. 2014;**9**:1-13

[90] Singh R, Khan NU, Singhal KC. *In vitro* antifilarial activity of *Sencio nudicaulis* Buch. Ham.—Effect on *Setaria cervi* (Nematoda Filarioidea). Indian Journal of Physiology and Pharmacology. 1996;**40**(3):231-236

[91] Saxena K, Dube V, Kushwaha V, Gupta V, Lakshmi M, Mishra S, et al. Antifilarial efficacy of *Hibiscus sabdariffa* on lymphatic filarial parasite *Brugia malayi*. Medicinal Chemistry Research. 2011;**20**(9):1594-1602

[92] Mathew N, Misra-Bhattacharya S, Perumal V, Muthuswamy K. Antifilarial lead molecules isolated from *Trachyspermum ammi*. Molecules. 2008; **13**(9):2156-2168

[93] Sashidhara KV, Singh SP, Misra S, Gupta J, Misra-Bhattacharya S. Galactolipids from *Bauhinia racemosa* as a new class of antifilarial agents against human lymphatic filarial parasite, *Brugia malayi*. European Journal of Medicinal Chemistry. 2012;**50**:230-235

[94] Singha M, Shakya S, Soni VK, Dangi A, Kumar N, Misra-Bhattacharya S. The n-hexane and chloroform fractions of *Piper betle* L. trigger different arms of immune responses in BALB/c mice and exhibit antifilarial activity against human lymphatic filarid *Brugia malayi*. International Immunopharmacology. 2009;**9**(6): 716-728

[95] Saini P, Gayen P, Nayak A, Kumar D, Mukherjee N, Pal BC, et al. Effect of ferulic acid from *Hibiscus mutabilis* on filarial parasite *Setaria cervi*: Molecular and biochemical approaches. Parasitology International. 2012;**61**(4): 520-531

[96] Gaur RL, Sahoo MK, Dixit S, Fatima N, Rastogi S, Kulshreshtha DK, et al. Antifilarial activity of *Caesalpinia bonducella* against experimental filarial infections. Indian Journal of Medical Research. 2008;**128**(1):65-70

[97] Al-Abd NM, Nor ZM, Mansor M, Hasan MS, Kassim M. Antifilarial and antibiotic activities of methanolic extracts of *Melaleuca cajuputi* flowers. Korean Journal of Parasitology. 2016; **54**(3):273-280

[98] Misra S, Verma M, Mishra SK, Srivastava S, Lakshmi V, Misra-Bhattacharya S. Gedunin and photogedunin of *Xylocarpus granatum* possess antifilarial activity against human lymphatic filarial parasite *Brugia malayi* in experimental rodent host. Parasitology Research. 2011;**109**: 1351-1360

[99] Sahare KN, Anandhraman V, Meshram VG, Meshram SU, Reddy MV, Tumane PM, et al. Anti-microfilarial activity of methanolic extract of *Vitex negundo* and *Aegle marmelos* and their phytochemical analysis. Indian Journal of Experimental Biology. 2008;**46**(2): 128-131

[100] Sahare KN, Singh V. *In-vitro* antifilarial activity of methanol extract of *Aegle marmelos*. Indo American Journal of Pharmaceutical Research. 2013;**3**(6):1-7

[101] Saini P, Mukherjee N, Mukherjee S, Roy P, Gayen P, Kumar D, et al. *Diospyros perigrena* bark extract induced apoptosis in filarial parasite *Setaria cervi* through generation of reactive oxygen species. Pharmaceutical Biology. 2015; **53**(6):813-823

[102] Ray AS, Joardar N, Mukherjee S, Rahaman CH, Babu SPS. Polyphenol

enriched ethanolic extract of *Cajanus scarabaeoides* (L.) Thouars exerts potential antifilarial activity by inducing oxidative stress and programmed cell death. PLoS One. 2018;**13**(12):e0208201

[103] Mishra V, Khan NU, Singhal KC. Potential antifilarial activity of fruit extracts of *Ficus racemosa* Linn. against *Setaria cervi in vitro*. Indian Journal of Experimental Biology. 2005;**43**:346-350

[104] Lakshmi V, Kumar R, Gupta P, Varshney V, Srivastava MN, Dikshit M, et al. The antifilarial activity of a marine red alga, *Botryocladia leptopoda,* against experimental infections with animal and human filariae. Parasitology Research. 2004;**93**:468-474

[105] Gupta J, Misra S, Mishra SK, Srivastava S, Srivastava MN, Lakshmi V, et al. Antifilarial activity of marine sponge *Haliclona oculata* against experimental *Brugia malayi* infection. Experimental Parasitology. 2012;**130**(4):449-455

[106] Lakshmi V, Srivastava S, Mishra SK, Misra S, Verma M, Misra-Bhattacharya S. In-vitro and in-vivo antifilarial potential of marine sponge, *Haliclona exigua* (Kirkpatrick) against human lymphatic filarial parasite *Brugia malayi*. Parasitology Research. 2009; **105**(5):1295-1301

[107] Lakshmi V, Misra-Bhattacharya S. Antifilarial activity of *Eucalyptus globulus Labill.* leaves against *Brugia malayi*. Bangladesh Pharmaceutical Journal. 2016;**19**:44-47

[108] Behera DR, Bhatnagar S. Assessment of macrofilaricidal activity of leaf extracts of *Terminalia* sp. against bovine filarial parasite *Setaria cervi*. Journal of Infection and Public Health. 2018;**11**(5):5643-5647

[109] Kushwaha V, Saxena K, Verma SK, Lakshmi V, Sharma RK, Murthy PK. Antifilarial activity of gum from *Moringa oleifera* Lam. on human lymphatic filaria *Brugia malayi*. Chronicles of Young Scientists. 2016;**2**:201-206

[110] Sahare KN, Anandharaman V, Meshram VG, Meshram SU, Gajalakshmi D, Goswami K, et al. *In vitro* effect of four herbal plants on the motility of *Brugia malayi* microfilariae. Indian Journal of Medical Research. 2008;**127**(5):467-471

[111] Deshmukh M, Sahare KN, Patidar RK, Mahajan B, Singh V. Antifilarial activity of *Butea monosperma* L. leaves extracts against *Setaria cervi*. Trends in Vector Research and Parasitology. 2014;**1**:1-5

[112] Shanmugapriya R, Ramnathan T. Antifilarial activity of seed extracts of *Ricinus communis* against *Brugia malayi*. Journal of Pharmacy Research. 2012; **5**(3):1448-1450

[113] Lakshmi V, Joseph SK, Srivastava S, Verma SK, Sahoo MK, Dube V, et al. Antifilarial activity *in vitro* and *in vivo* of some flavonoids tested against *Brugia malayi*. Acta Tropica. 2010;**116**(2):127-133

[114] Srinivasan L, Mathew N, Muthuswamy K. *In vitro* antifilarial activity of Glutathione S transferase inhibitors. Parasitology Research. 2009; **105**(4):1179-1182

[115] Casiraghi M, Anderson TJ, Bandi C, Bazzocchi C, Genchi CA. Phylogenetic analysis of filarial nematodes: Comparison with the phylogeny of *Wolbachia* endosymbionts. Parasitology. 2001;**122**:93-103

[116] Hoerauf A, Nissen-Pahle K, Schmetz C, Henkle-Duhrsen K, Blaxter ML, Buttner DW, et al. Tetracycline therapy targets intracellular bacteria in the filarial nematode *Litomosoides sigmodontis* and results in filarial infertility. Journal of Clinical Investigation. 1999;**103**:11-17

[117] Nuchprayoon S, Junpee A, Poovorawan Y. Random amplified polymorphic DNA (RAPD) for differentiation between Thai and Myanmar strains of *Wuchereria bancrofti*. Filaria Journal. 2007;**6**:6

[118] Ghedin E, Wang S, Spiro D, Caler E, Zhao Q, Crabtree J, et al. Draft genome of the filarial nematode parasite *Brugia malayi*. Science. 2007;**317**: 1756-1760

[119] Bennuru S, Meng Z, Ribeiro JM, Semnani RT, Ghedin E, Chan K, et al. Stage-specific proteomic expression patterns of the human filarial parasite *Brugia malayi* and its endosymbiont *Wolbachia*. Proceedings of the National Academy of Sciences of the United States of America. 2011;**108**:9649-9654

[120] Bhargavi R, Vishwakarma S, Murty US. Modeling analysis of GST (glutathione-s-transferases) from *Wuchereria bancrofti* and *Brugia malayi*. Bioinformation. 2005;**1**:25-27

[121] Acharya C, Coop A, Polli JE, Mackerell AD Jr. Recent advances in ligand-based drug design: Relevance and utility of the conformationally sampled pharmacophore approach. Current Computer-Aided Drug Design. 2011;**7**: 10-22

[122] Anderson AC. The process of structure-based drug design. Chemical Biology. 2003;**10**:787-797

[123] Allen FH, Taylor R. Research applications of the Cambridge structural database (CSD). Chemical Society Reviews. 2004;**33**:463-475

[124] Seiler KP, George GA, Happ MP, Bodycombe NE, Carrinski HA, Norton S. ChemBank: A small-molecule screening and cheminformatics resource database. Nucleic Acids Research. 2008; **36**:D351-D359

[125] Knox C, Law V, Jewison T, Liu P, Ly S, Frolkis A, et al. DrugBank 3.0: A comprehensive resource for 'omics' research on drugs. Nucleic Acids Research. 2011;**39**:D1035-D1041

[126] Li Q, Cheng T, Wang Y, Bryant SH. PubChem as a public resource for drug discovery. Drug Discovery Today. 2010;**15**:1052-1057

[127] Irwin JJ, Shoichet BK. ZINC: A free database of commercially available compounds for virtual screening. Journal of Chemical Information and Modeling. 2005;**45**:177-182

[128] Von Grotthuss M, Koczyk G, Pas J, Wyrwicz LS, Rychlewski L. Ligand: Info small-molecule meta-database. Combinatorial Chemistry & High Throughput Screening. 2004;7:757-761

Chapter 5

Nematode Infections Spread in Slovakia, an European Temperate Region

Ingrid Papajová and Jindřich Šoltys

Abstract

Nematode parasitic infections in the twenty-first century present a serious problem. They occur not only in developing but also in industrialised countries of temperate regions. It is well-known that these infections are common for communities living in poverty. Large numbers of nematode infections are transmitted via the faecal-oral route, where invasive parasitic eggs are excreted into the environments by the definitive hosts. The aim of this chapter is to investigate the occurrence of the most important nematode infections spread in major populations and population living under low hygienic standard conditions in the Slovak Republic territory. The data are compared with data available within European Union countries. The incidence of nematodes in domestic animals increases the health risks in low-privilege population. Contamination of the environment with nematodes as well as proposed countermeasures in urban and rural localities are discussed and suggested.

Keywords: nematodes, Slovakia, temperate region, environment

1. Introduction

Zoonoses are diseases transmitted by its natural way between man and animals pose a serious health risk. Principally, the zoonoses transmission is accomplished through close contact with domestic animals, especially dogs and cats, with whom we share more than 60 parasitic species [1]. Of about more than 370 parasite species, 40 of them are classified as zoonotic. According to the WHO data [2, 3], more than 2 billion people are affected by parasitic zoonoses. This is happening not only within developing but also in the industrialised countries, including Slovakia.

Zoonotic diseases are mainly transmitted through the soil or water. Primarily, they are represented by endoparasites such as protozoa and nematodes [4, 5]. In all of these diseases caused by endoparasites, the most likely route of man infection is oral transmission followed by the contact with infected humans and animals (wild, stray, and domestic), with contaminated food, soil, water, or infected environment. The main sources of the infected environment are faeces from infected animals living in close vicinity with the man. Though the contact with an animal is more intense in the rural than in the urban ecosystems, the likelihood of animal diseases spread is greater between stray animals or in animals without veterinary control.

The prevalence of intestinal parasitic diseases in Slovakia is due to its geographical location and relatively low good hygiene conditions. However, it may be easily dispensable in socially disadvantaged groups of people. Primarily, these diseases occur in the population of marginalised communities, which as a consequence of various factors are distinct by socio-economic exclusion. In Slovakia, according to the performed studies and governmentally released strategy papers, the group most at risk and living in poverty, which is socially excluded and discriminated, is represented by the Roma people. They are a very specific and the most numerous marginalised group in Slovakia [6]. The Roma population is the population with the progressive age structure, that is, with a high proportion of the younger population and with a low proportion of the population over the age of 60. Life expectancy, which is considered to be a fundamental indicator of the population's health status is within the Roma's men 55.3 and Roma's women 59.5 years, respectively. WHO specified the same numbers for the life expectancies in developing countries. The health status of Roma citizens is much worse when compared with the general (major) population. Particularly, there is a high risk of diseases linked with low hygiene standards. The most affected group are children, who are often exposed to the environmental and anthropogenic risks. Among of aformentioned parasitoses, the soil- and man-transmitted nematodes are the most important. They are represented by ascariasis (*Ascaris lumbricoides*), trichuriasis (*Trichuris trichiura*), ancylostomiasis (*Ancylostoma duodenale*), and necatoriasis (*Necator americanus*), which occur in a chronic form.

The objective of this chapter is to investigate: (i) the incidence of nematodes in domestic animals; (ii) contamination of the environment with nematodes; and (iii) the occurrence of the most important nematode infections spread in major populations and population living under low hygienic standard conditions in the Slovak Republic territory.

2. Material and methods

2.1 Coprological examination of excrements

Totally, 1237 dog faecal samples were collected and examined for the presence of parasite developmental stages. Dog faeces have been collected from around the dwellings, public places, or taken directly by the owners from backyards. After the collections, faecal samples were stored at 4°C and transferred to the laboratory for parasitological examination, which was performed within 24–48 h.

Flotation method with the sucrose flotation solution with specific density of 1.27 was used for coprological examination, where 3 g of faecal sample mixed with water was centrifuged for 5 min at 1200 rpm (Eppendorf 5804, Germany). After pouring out the supernatant, the sucrose flotation solution was added into the test tube. The sediment was then stirred and centrifuged again. After 5 min of sedimentation the test tube was refilled with flotation solution again. Than the top of tube was covered with cover glass to detect the eggs trapped in formed meniscus formed. All samples were further examined under the light microscope at 20× and 40× magnification (Leica Microsystems, DM 5000B light microscope, Germany).

2.2 Parasitological examination of soil samples

In order to identify the presence of parasites in the environment, totally 539 soil samples were collected within the vicinity of human settlements and around the kennels and dog pens. The sand samples were surveyed according to the Kazacos [7]. Briefly, 100 g of pooled sand sample, 100 ml of water, and 0.5 ml of Tween 40 were mixed and decanted for 10 min. Subsequently, the samples were sieved and replenished with 1000 ml of water. After 1 h sedimentation, the soil samples were centrifuged (Eppendorf 5804, Germany) and then floated with sucrose flotation solution (specific density of 1.3). Samples were examined under the light microscope at 20× and 40× magnification (Leica Microsystems, DM 5000B light microscope, Germany).

2.3 Parasitological examination of stool samples

Totally, 1571 children's stool samples were collected into the plastic containers. After an informed consent was signed by parents or legal guardians stool containers with unique identifiers were handed out together with the instruction regarding its return. Stool samples (up to 5–15 g of morning stool) were stored in refrigerator without any preservation at 4°C and transferred to the laboratory for examination that was performed within 24–48 h. Samples were examined with commercially available kit (Paraprep L, Mondial, France). Briefly, for each stool sample, 2 ml of ethyl acetate solution and 0.5 g of stool sample were added to 6 ml of 10% formalin in a mixing chamber. The chamber was then connected through filter with a conical collection chamber. Mixed content was incubated for 24 h at room temperature and the tube was centrifuged at 1000 rpm for 1 min (Eppendorf 5804, Germany). The entire samples volumes were collected into the collection chambers.

The supernatant was discarded and the sediment placed on microscope slides and covered with coverslip. The entire area was examined at 20× and 40× magnifications with Leica DM 5000B light microscope (Leica Microsystems, Germany).

2.4 Statistical analysis

Statistical significances were determined using Student t-test, ANOVA, and Dunnett Multiple Comparison test at the levels of significance 0.05, 0.01, and 0.001 (Statistica 6.0, USA) [8].

3. Results

3.1 Incidence of nematodes in dogs

All together, 1237 faeces samples from free living spaces and grass areas were collected within selected urban and rural ecosystems in the Slovak Republic territory for parasitological examinations. Endoparasites were found in 38.56% of all examined samples (**Table 1**). The most frequent were eggs from the family Ancylostomatidae (20.94%) and *Toxocara canis* (14.31%). Incidence of the other nematode eggs was confirmed in the following order: *Ascaris* spp. (8.08%),

Ecosystems	Negative	Positive	Number of samples	Prevalence (%)
Urban	580	198	778	25.45
Rural	133	89	222	40.09**
Low hygienic standard	46	191	237	80.59***
Overall prevalence	**760**	**477**	**1237**	**38.56**

Significance at the level P < 0.05.
****** *Significance at the level P < 0.01.*
******* *Significance at the level P < 0.001.*

Table 1.
Prevalence of parasitic developmental stages in dog faeces.

Trichuris vulpis (7.44%), *Toxascaris leonina* (5.58%), *Capillaria aerophila* (3.72%), strongyloid eggs (1.37%), and larvae of *Angiostrongylus vasorum* (0.40%; **Table 2**).

3.2 Nematode eggs occurrence in dog faeces in the urban ecosystem

Among of 1237 examined faecal specimens, 778 were collected within the urban ecosystem. Samples were collected randomly from the public spaces in seven cities of the Slovak Republic and examined microscopically. In summary, 25.45% of all samples were positive for the occurrence of parasitic nematodes (**Table 1**). Eggs, found in the excrements, were from the family Ancylostomatidae (8.61%), *T. canis* (8.10%), *T. leonina* (4.24%), *T. vulpis* (3.86%), *C. aerophila* (1.67%), and *Strongyloids* origin (1.80%; **Table 3**).

In 146 of positive faecal samples, a simple endoparasitic infection was the most common. Mixed infections with multiple intestinal parasites were detected in 52 cases. The most frequent was *T. canis* infection in combination with eggs from the family Ancylostomatidae, *T. leonina* and/or *T. vulpis* (30 samples). Fifteen samples contained three types of nematodes, where the most often infection was represented by helminths from the family Ancylostomatidae, *T. canis*, *T. leonina*, *C. aerophila*, and *T. vulpis*. Mixed infection consisting of four endoparasites was detected in seven samples. These cases were for the most part represented by the Ancylostomatidae family, *T. canis*, *T. leonina*, *C. aerophila*, and *T. vulpis* and/or *G. duodenalis*.

	Negative (n = 1237)	**Positive (n = 1237)**	**Prevalence (%)**
Toxocara canis	1060	177	14.31
Toxascaris leonine	1168	69	5.58
Ascaris spp.	1137	100	8.08
Ancylostomatidae *family*	978	259	20.94
Trichuris vulpis	1145	92	7.44
Capillaria aerophila	1191	46	3.72
Angiostrongylus vasorum	1232	5	0.40
Strongyloid eggs	1220	17	1.37

n, number of examined samples.

Table 2.
Occurrence of nematode eggs/larvae in dog faeces.

	Negative (n = 778)	**Positive (n = 778)**	**Prevalence (%)**
Toxocara canis	715	63	8.10
Toxascaris leonina	745	33	4.24
Ancylostomatidae family	711	67	8.61
Trichuris vulpis	748	30	3.86
Capillaria aerophila	765	13	1.67
Strongyloid eggs	764	14	1.80

n, number of examined samples.

Table 3.
Nematode eggs/larvae occurrence in dog faeces collected within urban ecosystem.

DOI: http://dx.doi.org/10.5772/intechopen.86389

3.3 Nematode eggs occurrence in dog faeces from rural ecosystem

Totally, 222 canine faeces samples were collected and coprologically examined from the rural ecosystem. Samples came from both, the public spaces and private land within numerous villages located in Slovakia.

The presence of parasitic intestinal developmental stages was confirmed in 40.09% of collected samples (**Table 1**), where 12 species of nematodes were detected. The most prevalent were the eggs of *T. canis* identified in 19.37% of cases and Ancylostomatidae family (16.67%). The other eggs present were *T. vulpis* (8.11%), *C. aerophila* (5.86%), *T. leonina* (0.45%), Strongyloid eggs (1.37%), and larvae of *A. vasorum* (1.44%; **Table 4**). Moreover, the dog faeces in rural areas contained also the eggs of non-specific parasites such as *Heterakis* spp., *Ascaridia* spp., *Moniezia* spp., and *Eimeria* spp. oocysts.

	Negative (n = 222)	Positive (n = 222)	Prevalence (%)
Toxocara canis	179	43	19.37
Toxascaris leonina	221	1	0.45
Ancylostomatidae family	185	37	16.67
Trichuris vulpis	204	18	8.11
Capillaria aerophila	209	13	5.86
Angiostrongylus vasorum	206	3	1.44
Strongyloid eggs	1220	17	1.37

n, number of examined samples.

Table 4.
Nematode eggs/larvae occurrence in dog faeces collected in rural ecosystem.

Parasitic monoinfection was detected in 58 samples. The most common was *T. canis* infection. Co-infection with two parasite species was observed in 17 cases, where the most common was *T. canis* and/or *T. vulpis* infection mixed with Ancylostomatidae and oocysts of *Isospora* spp. Combination of three endoparasites species was detected in nine samples. These mainly consisted of *T. canis*, *T. vulpis*, *C. aerophila*, and Ancylostomatidae eggs. Collection of four species was identified in three samples. Two samples contained a mixture of eggs similar to previous finding (Ancylostomatidae, *T. vulpis*, and *C. aerophila*), but in remaining samples *H. diminuta* eggs or oocysts *Hammondia/Neospora* spp. were also detected. One faecal sample contained eggs of the family Ancylostomatidae, *T. canis*, larvae of *A. vasorum* and *Sarcocystis* spp. oocysts. Joined co-infection with five endoparasites was found only in two samples (eggs of family Ancylostomatidae, *T. canis*, *T. vulpis*, *H. diminuta*, and *Isospora* spp. oocysts).

3.4 The occurrence of nematode eggs in dog faeces from areas with low environmental hygiene

In addition to the examination within standard urban and rural environment, the occurrence of parasitic eggs was determined in dog faces from areas with low environmental hygiene. Such locations in our region are represented by Roma settlements. Totally, 237 samples of dog faeces from four areas with low environmental hygiene were examined.

About 80.59% of canine faeces collected around houses were found to be positive for parasitic developmental stages (**Table 1**) and 13 different nematode species were identified. The most common findings were the eggs from the family Ancylostomatidae (65.40%). Despite the fact that the dogs are not host of *Ascaris* spp., the eggs of this nematode was very frequent (42.19%). Another nematodes present in dogs faeces were *T. canis, T. vulpis*, *T. leonina*, and *C. aerophila*. The occurrence of *A. vasorum* larvae was sporadic (**Table 5**).

Unlike in the urban and rural ecosystems, only 45 dogs living in areas with low hygiene environment have monoinfections. Multiple co-infections have been confirmed in 146 dogs. Two nematode species were detected in 48 samples and represented primarily by the eggs of the family Ancylostomatidae and *Ascaris* spp. Three nematode species were present in 43 samples, four in 29 samples, and five in 18 cases. Seven examined dogs were infected with six nematodes. Infection with seven nematodes (*T. canis*, *T. leonina*, *Ascaris* spp., Ancylostomatidae, *T. vulpis*, oocysts of *Isospora* sp., and *G. duodenalis*) were confirmed in one sample.

3.5 Contamination of soil by nematode eggs and larvae

The above average occurrence of nematode eggs and larvae in dog faeces poses high risk for environmental contamination. Therefore, their prevalence in the soil was monitored and its effect on population living in the affected areas was analysed.

Totally 539 samples of soil samples from cities in the Slovak Republic were examined to study the risk of environmental contamination. The presence of nematodes was confirmed in 14.47% of all samples. The representation for particular species was as follows: Ancylostomatidae family (7.79%), *Toxocara* spp. (7.24%), *Ascaris* spp. (3.71%), *T. leonina* (2.78%), *Trichuris* spp. (2.23%), and *Capillaria* spp. (0.37%).

In the cities, we focused primarily on the collection of samples from children's sandpits and public spaces. Together 497 samples were examined and the overall incidence of nematodes in urban environment was 9.86%. The most frequent eggs were of *Toxocara* spp. and eggs of family Ancylostomatidae. Randomly, the eggs of *T. leonina* and *Trichuris* spp. were detected (**Table 6**).

During the sandpits analysis, we sorted them as fenced and unfenced. The unfenced sandpits were found to be contaminated more than fenced. This finding was notable and statistically significant. In comparison with fenced sandpits (4.49%), the prevalence in unfenced sandpits was 12.32% (**Table 6**). The most frequent were the eggs of *Toxocara* spp. eggs from the Ancylostomatidae family. In

	Negative (n = 222)	Positive (n = 222)	Prevalence %
Toxocara canis.	166	71	29.96
Toxascaris leonina	202	35	15.77
Ascaris spp.	137	100	42.19
Ancylostomatidae family.	82	155	65.40
Trichuris vulpis	193	44	18.57
Capillaria aerophila	217	20	8.44
Angiostrongylus vasorum	235	2	0.84

n, number of examined samples.

Table 5.
Nematode eggs/larvae occurrence in dog faeces collected in localities with low hygienic standard.

addition, the unfenced sandpits comprised of *T. leonina*, *Trichuris* spp., and eggs from the family Ancylostomatidae (**Table 6**).

In rural environment, the soil samples were collected from parks, public spaces, and/or from private yards and gardens. In general, significantly higher incidence of parasitic eggs and larvae was found in soil samples collected from rural areas. Up to 44.44% of all examined samples were positive for the occurrence of Ancylostomatidae, *Toxocara* spp., as well as the *T. leonina* and *Trichuris* spp. eggs (**Table 7**).

The highest soil contamination was found in the areas with low environmental hygiene where up to 87.5% of the soil samples contained nematode eggs or larvae at various developmental stages (**Table 7**). The difference, when compared with rural and urban environment, was statistically significant. The soil collected from these sites was contaminated heavily with eggs of Ancylostomatidae family, *Ascaris* spp., *Toxocara* spp., *T. leonina*, and *Trichuris* spp. (**Table 7**).

The differences between the urban, rural and/or with low environmental hygiene examined sites were also compared according to the number of eggs detected per 100 g soil. Soil and sand samples in the urban ecosystem contained 1–10 eggs per 100 g sample. Typically, 1–20 eggs per 100 g sample were found in soil samples from the rural ecosystem. Soil samples collected in low-hygiene areas comprised of 10–1000 eggs per 100 g sample. Moreover, soil samples analysed at these sites contained in general up to 100–200 *Ascaris* spp. eggs per 100 g sample. Also, high numbers of nematode eggs were found for the family Ancylostomatidae (0–100 eggs per 100 g) and *Toxocara* spp. (0–50 eggs per 100 g).

	Sandpits (n = 497) % (p)	**Unfenced (n = 341) % (p)**	**Fenced (n = 156) % (p)**
Toxocara spp.	4.43 (22)	5.28 (18)	3.21 (5)
T. leonina	0.80 (4)	1.17 (4)	0
Ancylostomatidae family	3.62 (18)	4.69 (16)	1.28 (2)
Trichuris spp.	0.20 (1)	0.29 (1)	0
Overall prevalence	**9.86 (49)**	**12.32 (42)**	**4.49 (7)**

n, number of examined samples.

Table 6.
Nematode eggs occurrence in sandpits.

	Rural (n = 18) % (p)	**Rural with low hygienic standard (n = 24) % (p)**
Toxocara spp.	16.67 (3)	58.33 (14)
T. leonina	5.56 (1)	41.67 (10)
Ascaris spp.	0	79.17 (19)
Ancylostomatidae family	27.78 (5)	79.17 (19)
Trichuris spp.	5.56 (1)	41.67 (10)
Capillaria spp.	0	8.33 (2)
Overall prevalence	**44.44 (8)****	**87.50 (21)*****

n, number of examined samples; p, number of positive samples.
Significance at the level P < 0.05.
****Significance at the level P < 0.01.*
*****Significance at the level P < 0.001.*

Table 7.
Nematode eggs occurrence in rural environment and from localities with low hygienic standard.

3.6 Nematode spread in Slovak population

Parasitic nematodal disease incidence in the human population in correlation with environmental contamination and domestic animals was evaluated. Disease monitoring was focused on the most vulnerable children population divided into two groups. First one was represented by kids living satisfactory hygiene condition. Second one was represented by so-called marginalised group living in poor hygienic condition with limited access to the clean water. The living conditions in such settlements are often inadequate and the residents usually live in wooden or brick shacks that often lack basic infrastructural support. Under such conditions, the living space is often shared with a great number of dogs without appropriate veterinary care. As soon as the informed consent was signed by all participants, 1571 randomly selected stool samples from the major and minor (marginalised) population were collected and examined in collaboration with paediatricians and pertinent laboratories. The overall parasitic infections prevalence in children was 12.99%. The most dominant species were *A. lumbricoides* and *T. trichiura* (**Table 8**). *Hymenolepis nana* and *Hymenolepis diminuta* were detected sporadically. Despite the fact that no perianal examination was performed, *Enterobius vermicularis* eggs were present 26 faecal samples.

All examined children were divided into groups according to the environment where they live. The first group consisted of 851 children from the major population and came from the environment with standard hygiene conditions. The second, marginalised group consisted of 720 children who lived in an environment with low environmental hygiene.

Among of all 851 children who belong to the major population and lived in satisfactory hygiene conditions, only 5 kids were infected with *A. lumbricoides.* A totally different situation was observed in the so-called marginalised group, where the parasitoses incidence was up to 27.64% (**Table 8**).

A single parasitic monoinfection was observed in 170 children. Co-infection with two nematode species was found in 32 children. The most common infections were of *A. lumbricoides* and *T. trichiura*. Three kids were infected with *A. lumbricoides* and the single-cell parasite *G. duodenalis*. One child was infected with roundworm *A. lumbricoides* and *H. nana,* and one stool sample contained a combination of *T. trichiura* and *H. nana* eggs. Infection with three parasitic species was observed in two cases. The first was combination of *A. lumbricoides, T. trichiura*, and *G. duodenalis.* Second case consisted of combination with *T. trichiura* and *H. nana* and *G. duodenalis* cysts.

The incidence of nematodes in children at different ages was also examined. Based on the age, children were divided into three groups: Group 1: Newborn

	Total (n= 1571) % (p)	**Marginalised Roma population (n = 720) % (p)**	**Major non-Roma population (n = 851) % (p)**
Ascaris lumbricoides	12.03 (189)	25.56 (184)	0.59 (5)
Trichuris trichiura	2.99 (47)	6.53 (47)	0
Overall prevalence	**12.99 (204)**	**27.64 (199)*****	**0.59 (5)**

n, number of examined samples; p, number of positive samples.
Significance at the level P < 0.05.
***Significance at the level P < 0.01.*
****Significance at the level P < 0.001.*

Table 8.
Nematodes occurrence in children according the division to Roma or non-Roma population.

	Marginalised Roma population % (n/p)	Major non-Roma population % (n/p)
Newborn	14.17 (127/18)	0.94 (106/1)
Preschool age	29.66 (236/70)	0.63 (315/2)
School attending	28.10 (331/93)	0.48 (420/2)

n, number of examined samples; p, number of positive samples.

Table 9.
Nematodes occurrence in children according to age.

(0–2 years), Group 2: Preschool age (3–5 years), and Group 3: School age (6–18 years). The overall rejection rate between all participants due to incomplete data analysis or non-compliance was 15%.

In children from the marginalised group, the overall parasitic prevalence ranged from 14.17 to 29.66%. The least infected were kids under the age of 2. The most positive stool samples were found in preschool children and kids attending primary school. In opposite to the marginalised group, the overall disease prevalence in children living within major population did not exceed 1% (**Table 9**).

4. Discussion

At the present, it is necessary to create conditions for the co-existence of humans and animals. Man, in the course of domestication, incorporated various animal species into its environment. However, these animals can transfer and can be a source of many viral, bacterial, fungal, and parasitic diseases [9–11]. From this point of view, regarding the spread of parasitic diseases, a significant role is played by domestic animals. Especially, by the dogs and cats which share its living environment with humans. Thus, this co-habitation may represent an important source of contamination by parasites [12–14].

Parasitic status of house held dogs, as well as the other domestic animals, is affected by several factors such as the ecosystem type, breeding, wildlife, dogs use, age, and quality of veterinary care. In an urban ecosystem, the primary roles of the dog (hunting and protection) are diminishing, but its positive psychosocial and emotional influence on humans is on the rise. The town's infrastructure with flats and apartments impacts the ways how dogs are kept and share their living space with owners. Dogs in cities are in close contact with humans and became part of households. In some cases, the owner takes exaggerated care of their pets what leads to some kind of anthropomorphosis of domestic animals that occasionally could become family members' substitute [15, 16].

On the other side, such close contact can contribute to the contamination of the nearby human environment. For example, human toxocarosis is traditionally identified as a parasitic disease transmitted by contaminated soil. However, several studies have pointed out on the possibility of transfer through direct contact with the infected animal's fur. For instance, Wolfe and Wright [17] detected the eggs of *Toxocara* spp. on the coat of 25% examined dogs, where up to 4.20% of eggs were embryonated (capable of infection) and nearly 30% were still developing. Roddie et al. [18] detected *T. canis* eggs in 67% of dogs, and especially in puppies whose contact was limited to its own litter. An alarming discovery was that up to 82.4% of the eggs were viable and either embryonated or under development. In addition to the toxocara eggs, Wolfe and Wright [19] found in dog's fur, the eggs of *Nematodirus battus*, which usually do not parasite on dogs. It is likely that adult dogs have picked up the parasites from the other animal species in outside environment by rolling and playing on contaminated soil. Similar findings on the occurrence of infectious parasitic egg in the coat of various dog breeds were also confirmed by Aydenizöz-Özkayhan et al. [20]. The total prevalence of intestinal nematodes in urban localities in Slovakia was 25.45%. In dog excrements, we confirmed the eggs from family Ancylostomatidae, *T. canis*, *T. leonina*, *T. vulpis*, *C. aerophila,* and *Strongyloid* origin. Our results corresponded with those previously published by Antolová et al. [21] and Szabová et al. [22].

In rural ecosystems, the dogs have less companion function and are predominantly kept to guard properties. Usually, the animals do not have access to the interior spaces and are kept loosely on the yards or in the kennels. Under such conditions and in the case of infection, they can spread parasitic germs in surrounding territories. We found that in most municipalities there is no appropriate veterinary care, which may result in insufficient attention to the animal health. Additionally, this is probably also related with poor public health awareness and overall ignorance of the parasitic diseases spread associated with domestic animals. From various reasons, the dog health care very often does not include the prevention against parasitic diseases spread. Especially, in the animals that have no clinical symptoms, a visit to a local veterinarian is not necessary. Another phenomenon is free movement of dogs in villages what is the result of poorly maintained fences and also the owner's negligence. This leads to the spread of parasites into larger areas. The possibility of wandering and close uncontrolled contact with wildlife increases the probability of parasitic infections occurrence in domestic animals. Free living animals that are not under veterinary supervision may be an important source of infection. Many studies have confirmed that there is a higher parasitic of parasites in the population of dogs living in a rural ecosystem than in an urban ecosystem. Fok et al. [23] compared the occurrence of helminths in rural and urban dogs. A higher incidence of helminths was found in rural dogs (56%) when compared with cities (44%). Similar statistically significant difference in domestic animal parasitoses prevalence in the rural and urban ecosystem was reported also by Dubná et al. [24]. The total prevalence of parasites in municipalities around city Prague was 41.7%; meanwhile in the urban ecosystem, it was only 17.60%. Moreover, in a rural ecosystem, the authors found higher prevalence for all 13 detected species. Work of Habluetzel et al. [25] showed that 48.4% of dogs from the rural ecosystem had *T. canis* eggs, while only 26.2% of dogs were infected in the city. A slightly higher prevalence (40.6%) of parasitic eggs in dogs in a rural ecosystem in the Neuquén region of Argentina than in the urban ecosystem (33.4%) was found by Soriano et al. [26]. At the same time, the authors confirmed a statistically significant difference in the prevalence between cestodes and protozoa. In the rural ecosystem, *Taeniidae* ova were found in 44.7% of dogs and sporocysts of *Sarcocystis* spp. in 19.0% of dogs. The prevalence of these parasites in dogs did not exceed 3%. The prevalence of endoparasites in dogs from rural localities in Slovak Republic was 40.09%. *T. canis* and the eggs from family Ancylostomatidae appeared to be the most frequent. Similarly, Szabová et al. [22] confirmed endoparasites in 45.10% of dogs in Slovakia. Our results are similar to the records from neighbouring countries. In Poland, Borecka [27] found parasites in 34.20% of dog excrements and the most frequent were eggs from the family Ancylostomatidae. Dubná et al. [24] reported parasites in 41.7% of dogs examined in Czech Republic, where the most prevalent was *T. canis*.

Among the other important factors affecting the occurrence of parasites within human population is socio-economic status and environmental hygiene quality. In the developing countries, the domestic animals health care is not addressed properly. It is affected by unsatisfactory financial income in large proportion of the population, as well as with low level of health awareness and poor veterinary care. In Nigeria, Ugbomoiko et al. [28] detected 68%, predominantly of *T. canis*, intestinal parasites incidence. The high prevalence of toxocariasis in both dogs and humans was observed by Agudelo et al. [29] within the underprivileged districts of Bogota (Colombia).

Traub et al. [30] found that in Indian community with a low social status 99% of dogs were infected with at least one species of parasite. The most frequent eggs present in the faeces were of family Ancylostomatidae (94.0%), *A. lumbricoides* (31.0%), *T. trichiura* (25.0%), and *Isospora belli* oocysts (2.0%). The occurrence of typically human parasites in a dog's faeces points on the role of a dog as mechanical disseminators of parasitic germs. An increased incidence of parasites may also be found in socially deprived communities living in industrially well-developed countries. In our study, the total prevalence of intestinal parasites among dogs from the areas with low environmental hygiene was 80.59% and 13 different species with predominance of *Ascaris* spp. and family Ancylostomatidae were identified. Rudohradská et al. [31] reported a high parasitic incidence in dogs from segregated Roma settlements in Slovakia. The eggs of at least one parasite were detected in 73.8% of dog faeces samples. The risk of nematode parasites spread in ecosystems may also be increased by lack of owner's interest to perform regular antiparasitic treatment (dehelmintisation).

Increase in the number of dogs over the time in the cities with very limited access to green areas leads to the accumulation of excrement/faces in public spaces. The pollution of public spaces occurs despite the existence of laws (differs from country to country) regulating the conditions for housing and breeding the animals. For instance, in Slovakia, it is Act No. 282/2002 [32] and paragraph 6, which instructs the owners how to remove biological waste from the environment. The goal of law is to eliminate both factors: the negative aesthetic effect and removal of the endoparasites, which are released into the environment. In particular, dogs and cats are often infected with *Toxocara* spp. and are capable to initiate human toxocarosis. Activities related with the maintenance of urban vegetation, such as lawns and gardens care can contribute to the excrements and parasitic germs dispersal on large areas, where subsequent degradation of excrements leads to the spread parasitic propagative stages in the soil. Such contaminated land is source of further infection and reinfection of animals and poses critical risk to human health. The occurrence of endoparasitic developmental stages is monitored regularly by local health authorities. Mizgajska [33] shows that in Poland, soil contamination by endoparasites in urban development ranges between 38 and 53%, where the most frequent are *Toxocara* spp. and *Trichuris* spp. The high incidence of *Toxocara* spp. (67%) was also detected by Ruiz de Ybanez et al. [34] in the parks of Murcia (Spain). Somewhat lower level of soil contamination (45.5%) was observed by Martínez-Moreno et al. [35] in the urban parks of Cordoba, where *Toxocara* spp. and *T. leonina* were also detected.

Mizgajska-Wiktor and Jarosz (2007) performed a 5-year epidemiological monitoring for parasitic soil contamination in the city of Poznan and its surroundings. Interestingly, there was higher soil contamination within the city (19.8%) than in its rural area (15.6%). Gawor et al. [36] studied the epidemiology of soil contamination and the probability of reinfection in children diagnosed with toxocarosis. After the examination of soil around the households of sick children, it was found that *Toxocara* spp. occurred more frequently in rural settlements (27.5%) than in urban environment (21.1%).

An extensive attention should also be focused on the endoparasitic contamination of children's playgrounds where if not properly fenced the dogs and cats can litter. Children who have not yet developed their hygienic habits and are in direct contact with sand or may have geophagia are at the most risk. Ferre and Dorchies [37] detected *Toxocara* spp. on 38% of examined playgrounds and public parks in Toulouse (France). Talvik et al. [38] in Estonia found higher incidence of *Toxocara* spp. in sandpits (17.8%), which were contaminated by cat excrements, when compared with the soil in the parks (4.2%).

Our results confirmed that the occurrence of endoparasites at children's playgrounds is also affected by the level of protection against house held or free living animals. Jansen et al. [39] confirmed that fenced sandpits reduced the occurrence of parasitic developmental stages in comparison to the unprotected. This finding was endorsed by the study of Blaszkowska et al. [40] who carried out a survey on parasitic contamination in Lodz (Poland). Fenced sandpits and playgrounds, which were part of schools or kindergartens, contained only 1.4% geohelminths eggs. Meanwhile up to 15.7% of soil samples were found to be positive in unfenced playgrounds. The clear influence of fencing on the reduction of sand and soil contamination has also been confirmed by Dubná et al. [24] and Avcioglu and Balkaya [41].

As we mentioned earlier, younger population is most vulnerable to the nematode infections. Our results show that the total prevalence of nematodes within population with low hygiene standards was 27.64%, while only a small number of infections (0.59%) were observed within major population. *A. lumbricoides* was found to be the leading parasite (25.56%) and results corresponded with those of Rudohradská et al. [42]. Kubiak et al. [43] reported the prevalence of intestinal helminth infections among children in Poland from 3.30 to 46.30% where the most frequent parasite was *E. vermicularis.* In our study, *E. vermicularis* eggs were present in some stool samples. Since no perianal swabs were performed, only heavy infections could be detected. Significant differences in the nematodes prevalence between marginalised population and the major population were constantly confirmed. Based on our results, we can definitely conclude that nematode infections even now in twenty-first century still present a serious health problem.

5. Conclusion

Despite the temperate climatic conditions, nematode infections are still a threat to the public health. The counter measures against diseases spread should be engaged at several levels. Those are represented by appropriate sanitation, disruption of natural parasitic life cycles, soil decontamination, and improvement in hygiene standards. This all should be accomplished through the following actions:

- Perform compulsory surveys regarding the epidemiology, the presence of intermediate, and definitive hosts and soil contamination.

- Approaches such as geographical information systems (GIS) including spatial and environmental analysis should be considered and utilised to reveal biogeographical properties for particular parasitic diseases spread.

- Scrutinise the cultural and social habits from the rural and urban areas and examine the sanitary conditions and hygiene in affected areas.

- Implement appropriate control strategies, for the urban and rural settings, to protect farmers and pet owners.

- Increase public awareness about parasitic diseases spread via community centres, local governmental authorities, veterinary and health care services.

Acknowledgements

This work was supported by the grants VEGA no. 2/0125/17 (0.5) and APVV-18-0351 (0.5). We declare that we have no conflict of interest, and we have no financial or personal relationships with other people or organisations that could inappropriately influence our work. The proposal was reviewed and approved by the Ethical Commission of Institute of Parasitology SAS in Košice. Children's parents, legal representatives, agreed with all investigations and signed the informed consent prior to examinations and hospitalisations. We would like to thank people (students, postdocs, and colleagues) who allowed us to gather data needed for elaboration of this chapter.

Author details

Ingrid Papajová* and Jindřich Šoltys
Institute of Parasitology, Slovak Academy of Sciences, Košice, Slovak Republic

*Address all correspondence to: papaj@saske.sk

References

[1] Macpherson CNL. Human behaviour and the epidemiology of parasitic zoonoses. International Journal for Parasitology. 2005;**35**:1319-1331

[2] WHO—World Health Organization. Accelerating Work to Overcome the Global Impact of Neglected Tropical Diseases: A Roadmap for Implementation. Vol. 2012. Washington: WHO. pp. 1-42

[3] WHO. World Health Statistics 2014. Available from: http://apps.who.int/iris/bitstream/10665/112738/1/9789240692671_eng.pdf

[4] Bajer A. *Cryptosporidium* and *Giardia* spp. infections in humans, animals and the environment in Poland. Parasitology Research. 2008;**104**(1):1-17

[5] Cacciò SM, Ryan U. Molecular epidemiology of giardiasis. Molecular and Biochemical Parasitology. 2008;**160**(2):75-80

[6] Mušinka A, Škobla D, Hurrle J, Matlovičová K, Kling J. Atlas of Roma Communities in Slovakia 2013. Regional Centre for UN Developmental Programme for EU in Bratislava. Bratislava: UNDP; 2014

[7] Kazacos KR. Improved method for recovering ascarid and other helminth eggs from soil associated with epizootics and during survey studies. American Journal of Veterinary Research. 1983;**44**:896-900

[8] STATISTICA 6.0. USA: StatSoft Inc

[9] Irwin PJ. Companion animal parasitology: A clinical perspective. International Journal for Parasitology. 2002;**32**(5):581-593

[10] Macpherson, CNL, Meslin, FX, Wandeler AI. Dogs, Zoonoses and Public Health. Wallingford: CABI Publishing, 2000, pp. 382, ISBN 0-85199-436-9

[11] Robertson ID, Thompson RC. Enteric parasitic zoonoses of domesticated dogs and cats. Microbes and Infection. 2002;**4**(8):867-873

[12] Nareaho A, Puomio J, Saarinen K, Jokelainen P, Juselius T, Sukura A. Feline intestinal parasites in Finland: Prevalence, risk factors and anthelmintic treatment practices. Journal of Feline Medicine and Surgery. 2012;**14**(6):378-383

[13] Nikolic A, Dimitrijević S, Bobić B. Canine giardiosis in an urban area: A possible source on infection of man. The journal of Protozoology Research. 2001;**11**(3-4):61-65

[14] Robertson ID, Irwin PJ, Lymbery AJ, Thompson RCA. The role of companion animals in the emergence of parasitic zoonoses. International Journal for Parasitology. 2000;**30**(12):1369-1377

[15] Albert A, Bulcroft K. Pets and urban life. Anthrozoos: A Multidisciplinary Journal of The Interactions of People & Animals. 1987;**1**(1):9-25

[16] Power E. Furry families: Making a human–dog family through home. Social & Cultural Geography. 2008;**9**(5):535-555

[17] Wolfe A, Wright IP. Human toxocariasis and direct contact with dogs. Veterinary Record: Journal of the British Veterinary Association. 2003;**152**(14):419-422

[18] Roddie G, Stafford P, Holland C, Wolfe A. Contamination of dog hair with eggs of *Toxocara canis*. Veterinary Parasitology. 2008;**152**(1-2):85-93

[19] Wolfe A, Wright IP. Parasitic nematode eggs in fur samples from

dogs. Veterinary Record: Journal of the British Veterinary Association. 2004;**154**:408-409

[20] Aydenizöz-Özkayhan M, Yağci BB, Erat S. The investigation of *Toxocara canis* eggs in coats of different dog breeds as a potential transmission route in human toxocarosis. Veterinary Parasitology. 2008;**152**:94-100

[21] Antolová D, Reiterová K, Miterpáková M, Stanko M, Dubinský P. Circulation of *Toxocara* spp. in suburban and rural ecosystems in the Slovak Republic. Veterinary Parasitology. 2004;**126**(3):317-324

[22] Szabová E, Juriš P, Miterpáková M, Antolová D, Papajová I, Šefčíková H. Prevalence of important zoonotic parasites in dog populations from the Slovak Republic. Helminthologia. 2007;**44**(4):170-176

[23] Fok E, Szatmári V, Busák K, Rozgonyi F. Epidemiology: Prevalence of intestinal parasites in dogs in some urban and rural areas of Hungary. Veterinary Quarterly. 2001;**23**(2):96-98

[24] Dubná S, Langrová I, Nápravník J, Jankovská I, Vadlejch J, Pekár S, et al. The prevalence of intestinal parasites in dogs from Prague, rural areas, and shelters of the Czech Republic. Veterinary Parasitology. 2007;**145**(1-2):120-128

[25] Habluetzel A, Traldi G, Ruggieri S, Attili AR, Scuppa P, Marchetti R, et al. An estimation of *Toxocara canis* prevalence in dogs, environmental egg contamination and risk of human infection in the Marche region of Italy. Veterinary Parasitology. 2003;**113**(3-4):243-252

[26] Soriano SV, Pierangeli NB, Roccia I, Fabian H, Bergagna J, Lazzarini LE, et al. A wide diversity of zoonotic intestinal parasites infects urban and rural dogs in Neuquen, Patagonia, Argentina. Veterinary Parasitology. 2010;**167**:81-85

[27] Borecka A. Differentiation of *Toxocara* spp. eggs isolated from the soil by PCR-linked RFLP. Helminthologia. 2004;**41**:185-187

[28] Ugbomoiko US, Ariza L, Heukelbach J. Parasites of importance for human health in Nigerian dogs: High prevalence and limited knowledge of pet owners. BMC Veterinary Research. 2008;**4**(1):e49

[29] Agudelo C, Villareal E, Cáceres E, López C, Eljach J, Ramírez N, et al. Human and dogs *Toxocara canis* infection in a poor neighborhood in Bogota. Memórias do Instituto Oswaldo Cruz. 1990;**85**(1):75-78

[30] Traub RJ, Robertson ID, Irwin P, Mencke N, Thompson RA. The role of dogs in transmission of gastrointestinal parasites in a remote tea-growing community in northeastern India. The American Journal of Tropical Medicine and Hygiene. 2002;**67**(5):539-545

[31] Rudohradská P, Papajová I, Juriš P. Pets as a source of parasitic soil contamination in the settlements of marginalised groups of inhabitants. Folia Veterinaria. 2011;**55**(1):33-35

[32] Act No. 282/2002. On breeding and keeping of pets in the Slovak Republic

[33] Mizgajska H. Eggs of *Toxocara* spp. in the environment and their public health implications. Journal of helminthology. 2001;**75**(2):147-151

[34] Ruiz de Ybanez MRR, Garijo MM, Alonso FD. Prevalence and viability of eggs of *Toxocara* spp. and *Toxascaris leonina* in public parks in eastern Spain. Journal of Helminthology. 2001;**75**:169-173

[35] Martínez-Moreno FJ, Hernández S, López-Cobos E, Becerra C, Acosta I,

Martínez-Moreno A. Estimation of canine intestinal parasites in Córdoba (Spain) and their risk to public health. Veterinary Parasitology. 2007;**143**(1):7-13

[36] Gawor J, Borecka A, Zarnowska H, Marczyńska M, Dobosz S. Environmental and personal risk factors for toxocariasis in children with diagnosed disease in urban and rural areas of Central Poland. Veterinary Parasitology. 2008;**155**:217-222

[37] Ferre P, Dorchies P. Prevalence of *Toxocara* spp. eggs in sandpits of eight public parks in Toulouse (SW France). Revue de Médecine Vétérinaire. 2000;**151**:501-506

[38] Talvik H, Moks E, Mägi E, Järvis T, Miller I. Distribution of *Toxocara* infection in the environment and in definitive and paratenic hosts in Estonia. Acta Veterinaria Hungarica. 2006;**54**(3):399-406

[39] Jansen J, Van Knapen F, Schreurs M, Van Wijngaarden T. *Toxocara* ova in parks and sand-boxes in the city of Utrecht. Tijdschrift voor diergeneeskunde. 1993;**118**(19):611-614

[40] Blaszkowska J, Wojcik A, Kurnatowski P, Szwabe K. Geohelminth egg contamination of children's play areas in the city of Lodz (Poland). Veterinary Parasitology. 2013;**192**(1-3):228-233

[41] Avcioglu H, Balkaya İ. The relationship of public park accessibility to dogs to the presence of *Toxocara* species ova in the soil. Vector-Borne and Zoonotic Diseases. 2011;**11**(2):177-180

[42] Rudohradská P, Halánová M, Ravaszová P, Goldová M, Valenčáková A, Halán M, et al. Prevalence of intestinal parasites in children from minority group with low hygienic standards in Slovakia. Helminthologia. 2012;**49**(2):63-66

[43] Kubiak K, Wrońska M, Dzika E, Dziedziech M, Poźniak H, Leokajtis M, et al. The prevalence of intestinal parasites in children in preschools and orphanages in the Warmia-Masuria province (North-Eastern Poland). *Przegląd* epidemiologiczny. 2015;**69**:483

Section 4

Helminthes and Livestock

Chapter 6

Anthelmintic Resistance in Livestock

Morutse Mphahlele, Nthatisi Molefe, Ana Tsotetsi-Khambule and Thekisoe Oriel

Abstract

For decades anthelmintics have been used as the primary control measure for worm infections in livestock. However, there has been continuous development of anthelmintic resistance (AR) by the parasitic worms infecting livestock. This chapter reviews AR in livestock with a special focus on treatment and control, modes of action of different anthelmintic classes, risk factors leading to development of AR, conventional and molecular tools used to detect AR, FAMACHA© and holistic control strategy to control anthelmintic resistance.

Keywords: anthelmintic resistance, helminths, livestock, benzimidazoles, imidazothiazoles, macrocyclic lactones

1. Helminths infecting livestock

Livestock can be infected with a variety of helminths on pastures, through ingestion of the larvae of the parasites on the contaminated grass, the most common of which are gastrointestinal nematodes and flukes [1]. It goes without saying that helminths have constantly been problematic and without doubt a long-standing concern that threatens the livestock industry [2] given that these parasites have a negative impact on animal productivity and welfare, affecting among other things feed intake, growth rate and milk yield [3]. Parasitic worms include tapeworms, roundworms, lungworms, liver flukes, ring worms, hook worms and whip worms. Transmission of GIT parasites is fairly direct in most cases; the infective eggs or oocyst are passed with the faeces when the animal defecates, the next animal would be infected if they graze in the contaminated areas, and humans could be infected through ingestion of contaminated food and water and/or through close interactions of humans with the infected animals [4]. The annual cost associated with parasitic diseases has been estimated at 1 billion dollars in Australia [5], 7.11 billion dollars in Brazil [6], and believed to be tens of billions of dollars worldwide [5].

2. Treatment and control

2.1 Chemotherapy

Worm control in most farms is exclusively based on anthelmintic treatments rather than on management practices that embraces integrated strategies. The currently available anthelmintics belong to different drug classes, i.e. macrocyclic lactones (MLs), benzimidazoles (BZs), tetrahydropyrimidines-imidazothiazoles, aminoacetonitrile derivatives (AADs) and spiroindoles. The compounds of these drug classes are potent against a broad range of nematode species, and, furthermore, MLs are effective against many arthropod parasites, whilst BZs also versus some flat worm species [7]. However, even with correct administration of treatment, figures point that the use of anthelmintics is still an expensive way of controlling parasitic diseases [5].

2.2 Modes of action of different anthelmintic classes

Each class of anthelmintics has a unique mode of action against parasites [8]. Imidazothiazoles (IM), such as levamisole, are acetylcholine agonists that act on the nervous system of the parasite [8]. These drugs cause muscle contraction and paralysis in the helminth, resulting in the eventual expulsion of the parasite from the body [9]. Macrocyclic lactones, on the other hand, act on glutamate-gated chloride channels (GluCl) causing paralysis of the parasite neuromusculature, including the pharynx, thereby preventing the worm from feeding [8]. The target of benzimidazoles is, however, the tubulin within the parasite intestinal cells, which forms into microtubules that are necessary for nutrient acquisition [10]. Benzimidazoles bind to the β-tubulin component preventing it from forming microtubules within the intestinal cells of the helminth. This impairs the uptake of nutrients and prevents the transportation of necessary digestive enzymes resulting in death due to starvation [9]. Additional effects of benzimidazoles on nematodes include depletion of energy reserves and the inhibition of waste excretion [11]. The only available aminoacetonitrile derivative on the market today is monepantel [11]. It acts as an agonist of the mptl-1 channel, a channel belonging to a class of nicotinic acetylcholine receptors in the process causing constant fluctuation in muscle ions leading to muscle depolarisation and irreversible nematode paralysis [11]. Benzimidazoles and macrocyclic lactones are effective against the adult and immature stages of the parasite, whilst the imidazothiazoles are effective against the adults and the later stages of immature larvae [8]. In short, these drugs enter the worm and interact with its target receptor in order to trigger a harmful physiological effect [12]. **Figure 1** shows a schematic

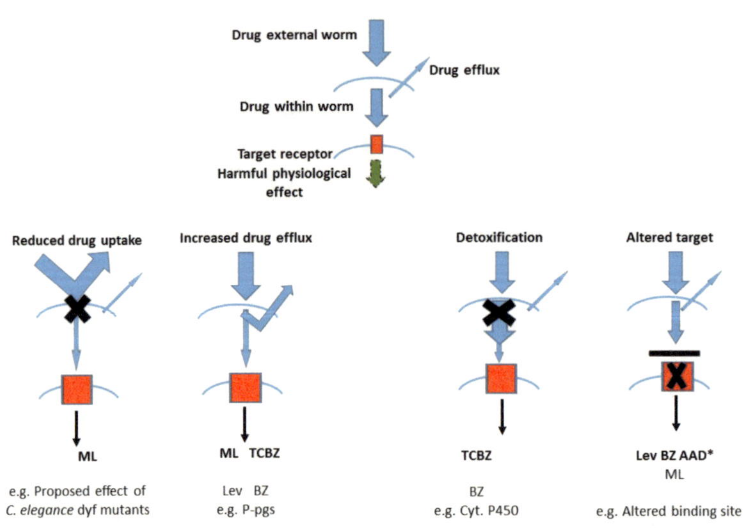

Figure 1.
Schematic representation of principally known anthelmintic resistance pathways and their relevance to each of the current anthelmintic drug classes [8].

representation of principally known anthelmintic resistance (AR) pathways and their relevance to each of the current anthelmintic drug classes.

The classes of broad-spectrum anthelmintics range from benzimidazoles, imidazothiazoles/tetrahydropyrimidines and macrocyclic lactones, but salicylanilides, phenolic substitutes and organophosphates are also popular [13]. Broad-spectrum anthelmintics are more commonly used in ruminants because they are capable of eliminating large numbers of parasites, besides being of easy administration and safe to the hosts [14].

3. Anthelmintic resistance

For decades anthelmintics have been used as the primary control measure for nematode parasites in sheep [15]. However, over the years there has been continuous and significant development of AR by the parasitic worms infecting livestock. Anthelmintic resistance can be defined as the ability of parasites to survive doses of drugs that would normally kill parasites of the same species and stage. It is inherited and selected for because the survivors of treatments pass genes for resistance onto their offspring. These resistant genes are initially rare in the population or arise as rare mutations, but as selection continues, their proportion in the population increases as does the proportion of resistant parasites [16].

Earlier work evaluated the knowledge that defined resistance in the year 1980, and from their study, they predicted the spread and future impact of resistance and also set goals for future research [17]. The earliest report of AR was in 1964 for *H. contortus* resistance to benzimidazole in treated sheep and was also the first for a modern drug in production animals [18]. Within 10 years of the first report of AR, resistance was found regularly in sheep parasites, followed by reports of resistance in horse and cattle nematodes [19]. Although anthelmintics have been efficient and work quickly, nematodes have developed resistance in a number of sheep-producing countries such as Australia [20], South Africa [21], New Zealand, [22], Switzerland [23] and Italy [24]. To this end the highest resistance has been observed with ivermectin (Ivomec®) and albendazole (Valbazen®) or fenbendazole (Safeguard® or Panacur®), and low to moderate resistance has been observed with levamisole (Levasole®, Tramisol®). Resistance to moxidectin (Cydectin®) is also prevalent and on the rise on many livestock farms [25]. In Africa, anthelmintic resistance has been reported in both the commercial and resource-poor farming sectors in at least 13 countries, and, among the commercial farms in South Africa, the situation is considered the worst in the world, with high levels of *Haemonchus contortus* resistance to all classes of anthelmintics [26].

Resistance to the two newer classes, the aminoacetonitrile derivatives and paraherquamide derivatives, is expected to follow [27]. There are anthelmintics still available, but multiple drug-resistant helminth strains have quickly developed, and producers and animal health professionals must now seek alternative methods of treatment and prevention [28]. Below are some prominent cases of anthelmintic resistance reported in the world (**Table 1**).

Sadly, anthelmintic resistance is now considered the status quo in most sheep-producing countries of the world [45], and repeated cross-sectional studies in Europe and South America have shown a worsening situation, with both multidrug and multispecies resistance which are increasingly more common [46, 47]. Although it is not widespread, resistance has already developed to two new active ingredients, monepantel and derquantel. This was despite spiroindole—derquantel—being marketed as a combination product to slow the development of resistance [48]. All of these highlight the urgent need to identify risk factors associated with AR development, to inform future recommendations on sustainable parasite control [49].

Country	Anthelmintic (class)	Nematode genera	Year AR reported	References
South Africa	Levamisole, morantel	*Trich/Tel* spp.	1990	[29]
South Africa	Benzimidazole, fenbendazole, rafoxinide, levamisole (BZ, SCL, IMID)	*Haemonchus* spp.	1992–1996	[30]
South Africa	Albendazole, closantel, ivermectin, levamisole (BZ, SCL, AVM, IMID)	*Haemonchus* spp., *Trich/Tel* spp. and *Oesophagostomum* spp.	2003 and 2013	[31, 32]
Zimbabwe	Fenbendazole, albendazole, oxfendazole, levamisole (BZ, IMID)	*Haemonchus* spp., *Cooperia* spp.	1997 and 2003	[33, 34]
Zimbabwe	Fenbendazole, levamisole, rafoxanide (BZ, IMID, SCL)	*Haemonchus* spp.	1997	[35]
Zambia	Ivermectin, albendazole (AVM, BZ)	*Haemonchus* spp.	2001	[36]
Kenya	Ivermectin, fenbendazole (AVM, BZ)	*Haemonchus* spp., *Trich/Tel* spp. and *Oesophagostomum* spp.	1995	[37]
Germany	Levamisole, ivermectin (IMID, AVM)	*Trich/Tel* spp.	2012	[38]
Norway	Albendazole (BZ)	*Trich/Tel* spp.	2012	[39]
Northern Ireland	Benzimidazole, moxidectin, avermectin, levamisole (BZ, MLB, AVM, IMID)	*Trich/Tel* spp., *Cooperia* spp.	2013	[40]
Switzerland	Avermectin (AVM)	*Haemonchus* spp., *Trich/Tel* spp.	2007	[41]
Brazil	Ivermectin (AVM)	*Haemonchus* spp.	2013	[42]
India	Fenbendazole, benzimidazole, thiabendazole, tetramisole (BZ, IMID)	*Haemonchus* spp., *Trich/Tel* spp.	2013, 2011	[43], [44]

BZ, benzimidazoles; ML, macrocyclic lactones (AVM, avermectines, or MLB, milbemycin); nicotinic agonists (IMID, imidazothiazoles, or TETR, tetrahydropyrimidines); AAD, aminoacetonitrile derivatives; SCL, salicylanilides; Tel, Teladorsagia; Trich, Trichostrongylus

Table 1.
Some cases of anthelmintic resistance.

4. Risk factors for development of AR

The control of gastrointestinal parasitism for small ruminants has long been under threat from the development of anthelmintic resistance by parasite populations [46]. However, in recent years it has become evident that this is also an emerging problem for cattle [50]. Resistance against drugs belonging to the same anthelmintic drug class is called side resistance, whereas cross and multidrug resistance refer to resistance against two or multiple drugs belonging to different anthelmintic drug classes [47]. Development of AR can be limited by ensuring that the parasites are exposed to an effective drug dose and to consider the timing and frequency of anthelmintic drug treatments so that only a small proportion of the population is exposed to the anthelmintic [51]. The main factors for the selection for anthelmintic resistance are high-treatment frequency, [52] underdosing and the use of the same anthelmintic class over several years [48]. These factors, individually or in combination, together with the risk of underdosing and continued use of one class of anthelmintics, irrespective of efficacy status are frequently encountered factors enhancing development of anthelmintic resistance [53]. Underestimation of real weight has a potential to lead to underdosing, which can contribute to the development of AR [48]. The results of a South African study attributed AR observed in goats to underdosing caused by visual appraisal of an animal to estimate its weight as opposed to the actual weighing before dosing to determine the correct anthelmintic dosage [31]. In consideration of ensuring a correct dose, livestock farmers have to determine the weight as accurately as possible, preferably by individually weighing each animal [40]. Alternatively, the use of a heart girth measurement tape is also recommended as this would certainly provide small-scale farmers with a practical tool to be used in determining the live weight of their small stock [54]. The use of faecal egg count reduction tests (FECRT) and egg hatch assays in combination with morphological identification of third-stage larvae recovered from pre- and post-treatment cultures may provide a solid indication of the presence of anthelmintic resistance.

5. Anthelmintic resistance monitoring

5.1 Faecal egg count reduction test

The faecal egg count reduction test is the main method of detection of anthelmintic resistance in nematodes of veterinary importance [55]. In the FECRT, populations of gastrointestinal nematodes of sheep are considered susceptible when drug efficacy exceeds 95% (reduction in FECRT). Conversely, resistance is present when efficacy is <95%. The equivalent efficiency benchmark for resistance is 90% for other host species. However, reductions in efficacy require interpretation in the light of different situations [56], where, for instance, the 95% cutoff is more complex than it seems because some drugs have very high efficacy (99.9%) against some parasite species but lower (say, 95%) for others in the same host. FECRT is an in vivo method that involves the nematodes in the sheep as the experimental unit [57–59]. An advantage of FECRT is that it can be used with all groups of anthelmintics that are available today. The disadvantage is that the faecal egg count (FEC) levels do not always correspond to the number of adult worms inside the animals. However, FECs in young sheep correlate fairly well to the burden of adult worms, at least compared to the situation in adult sheep [58, 59]. Furthermore, the FECRT can only detect AR if there are over 25% of resistant nematodes in a population and also requires a large number of sheep and is therefore difficult to be used in small flocks [58, 59]. Whilst FECRT has been used for over 30 years, more recent work has revealed shortcomings in the diagnosis of resistance based on proportional reduction. The problem is that diagnosis overestimates resistance when it is emerging. A study by Lyndal-Murphy [60] reported on the use of statistical simulation studies to consider situations for sheep where resistance is defined as <95% efficacy. This study has shown that FECRT results too often diagnose resistance where it does not exist. FECRT has been used successfully to detect AR in many other countries including Zimbabwe [33], Zambia [36], Brazil [42], Kenya [37] and Switzerland [41].

5.2 Egg hatch test

Egg hatch test (EHT) is an in vitro test that can be used to measure AR [61]. EHT can only measure BZ resistance. In practice, fresh eggs are either diluted in increasing concentrations of thiabendazole (TBZ) or diluted in a predetermined concentration (discriminating dose) and incubated for 48 hours. The eggs hatched are then counted under an inverted microscope. Discriminating doses have been established in nematode species such as *H. contortus*. A discriminating dose is the dose required to prevent hatching of 99% of susceptible eggs. The EHT can detect resistance if there are at least 2–3% resistant eggs [58].

Egg hatch test and other in vitro tests generate dose-response lines [10]. This allows the calculation of parameters, such as the concentration that kills 95% of eggs (the EC95), a single parameter used to compare isolates. Resistant worms will have a higher EC95 because a higher drug concentration is required to kill them. Such assays are underutilised tools for measuring resistant phenotypes. However, they have been fundamental tools for studying the results of experimental genetic crosses [62].

5.3 Larval development assay

Two versions of larval development test are used. The first was described in detail by Hubert and Kerbouf in 1992 [63]. The counted number of eggs in a 0.5 mL of egg suspension is put into each well in a 96-microtitre plate. The contents of the wells are then mixed, and the plates placed in an incubator under humidified conditions at 27°C for 48 hours for incubation of the eggs. After 48 hours, thiabendazole is added to the plates containing the egg suspension. The plates are incubated for 5 days; after which they will be examined to determine the survival of the larvae at different concentrations. All the L_3-stage larvae in each well must be counted, and the percentage inhibition of larval development is calculated using the formula [64]:

$$E = \frac{(\text{Eggs} + \text{L1}) - \text{L1}}{\text{Eggs} + \text{L1}} \times 100 \qquad (1)$$

In the second version, the micro-agar larval development test (MALDT) is performed as described by Coles et al. [57]. This test is also performed on 96-microtitre well plates. Stock solutions of thiabendazole/levamisole are prepared by predissolving the drugs in dimethyl sulfoxide (DMSO) with subsequent dilution in distilled water (1:4). Nematode eggs recovered from faecal samples are incubated for 7 days at 27°C in 96-well microtitre plates with the drug solution. The plates will normally have a culture medium (yeast extract with Earle's balanced salt solution and physiologic salt solution) in an aquatic solution of various concentrations of thiabendazole/levamisole and the determined proportion of nematode eggs in each well. After 7 days, the numbers of unhatched eggs and L_1–L_3 larvae in each well are counted under an inverted microscope. The rate of L_3 development in the discriminating dose (0.02 and 0.5 μg/ml for thiabendazole and levamisole, respectively) compared to the control is then used to determine if resistance is present; thus, the number of larvae developing from L_1 to L_3 stage in the discriminating dose of 0.02 μg/ml thiabendazole and 0.5 μg/ml levamisole is a clear indication of resistance.

5.4 Use of molecular techniques for AR monitoring

Nowadays, the traditional parasitological diagnostic techniques involving mainly microscopy have been complemented by a variety of new techniques and tools, mostly molecular in nature. To date, traditional methods are still routinely used despite the fact that they can be labour and time intense to perform [25]. PCR-based procedures have been proven to have greater sensitivity and specificity than 'conventional' diagnostic approaches reliant on microscopy and/or immune detection [65]. Studies with other models of resistance to xenobiotics demonstrated that migration plays a fundamental role in such things as the dispersion of insecticide-resistant genes in mosquitoes [66] and of antibiotic resistance among some species of bacteria [67]. There have been studies on the origin of the BZ-resistant alleles in worm populations. For instance, using RFLP studies on the isotype 1-tubulin gene, it was established that there are various BZ-resistant alleles in different resistant populations of *H. contortus* [68]. Using the same approach on two BZ-resistant populations, it was also found that the BZ-resistant alleles were probably already present in two *H. contortus* populations before this class of drugs was even developed [69].

6. FAMACHA© and targeted selective treatment

With nematode resistance now present to all three of the broad-spectrum anthelmintic classes (benzimidazoles, levamisole and macrocyclic lactones) used on ruminants [52], control strategies aiming to sustain effective parasitic control are of key importance. Methodologies designed to maintain refugia which are the size of the unselected proportion of the nematode population can help to reduce the build-up of resistance by preserving susceptible nematode genotypes which helps to dilute the frequency of resistance alleles and maintain anthelmintic efficacy [70].

One strategy that aims to achieve this is targeted selective treatment (TST), which involves the treatment of selected individuals that require treatment as opposed to treatment of the entire group [71]. Individuals are generally identified as needing to receive treatment on the basis of their level of parasitism [3]. Although TST strategies have been developed and applied successfully in sheep, there are considerably fewer studies on cattle, with the first insights into the application of TST having occurred relatively recently [72]. As there are important differences in host-parasite interactions and parasite epidemiology between cattle and sheep, differences in the methodology and application of TST in cattle can be expected. Although TST strategies in sheep have been shown to be beneficial in reducing selection for anthelmintic resistance [72], it is difficult to know which of the various strategies would be most effective under various scenarios. At present there are no direct comparisons of TST strategies in cattle, in part due to difficulties arising from confounding variables [72].

Simulation modelling on the other hand may offer an effective alternative and be highly beneficial in assessing the feasibility of novel control strategies. In the FAMACHA© system, operators assess the severity of parasitism by using a conjunctival colour chart which correlates to anaemia to choose affected animals for selective treatment. FAMACHA© was developed by a South African veterinarian, and it stands for Faffa Malan Chart. The application of FAMACHA© has been a pivotal example of a practical approach in managing resistance, as targeted treatment provides many potential benefits. One benefit is that it helps in the removal of worms from the most severely infected and affected animals and so reduces production losses in the most impacted animals. These animals also shed more eggs than other animals, so targeted treatment of a small proportion of the flock reduces a large proportion of pasture contamination. Most importantly, it reduces selection by reducing chemical use and maintaining refugia.

7. Holistic control strategy to control anthelmintic resistance

General risk factors for the development of AR in livestock include overuse of anthelmintics, underdosing, frequent movement and transfer of animals from one area to another and poor pasture management. Techniques such as body condition scoring, faecal egg detection, larval detection and FAMACHA© are still relatively underutilised when in combination with the use of anthelmintics. We propose that countries must develop integrated holistic system that will be a combined effort between animal health professionals, extension officers, farmer unions and drug companies where education is one of the most important components for helminthosis control and prevention of AR development (**Figure 2**). Farmers, both at large-scale commercial and small-scale communal farming, need to be constantly conscientised on the proper use of anthelmintics, pasture management and purchase and transportation of livestock from one area to another.

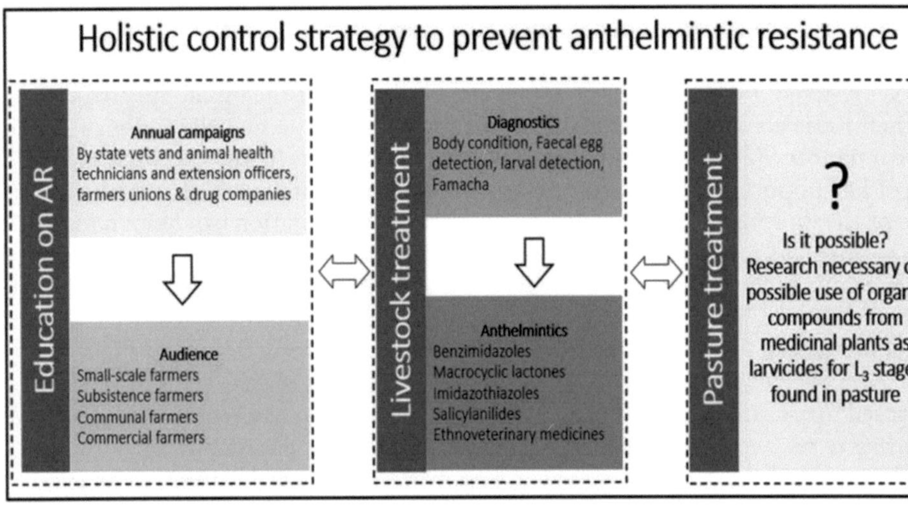

Figure 2.
A holistic AR prevention strategy which includes annual education campaigns to all types of farmers and application of different diagnostic techniques which then dictates necessary anthelmintic treatment.

Direct anthelmintic-like effects have been demonstrated in in vitro assays, which have shown that incubation in crude condensed tannin extracts reduced the development, viability, motility and migratory ability of parasite larvae [73]. Whilst there will be continuous development of synthetic compounds which will be used as anthelmintics, there is a need for increased scientific studies of conversion and adoption of natural compounds extracted from medicinal plants as a substantial number of them has been reported to contain anthelmintic activity [74]. Future research should also focus on possible treatment of pasture with organic compounds from medicinal plants in an attempt to control the larval stages of helminths.

8. Perspective (future control and prevention methods, necessary research)

Many of the approaches that are available for prevention of AR are still being researched and evaluated, and most of them are at present not suitable for the communal grazing systems of many resource-poor farmers; therefore, further research must still be conducted to ensure adaptability to both commercial and resource-poor farming operations. Another challenge facing both the farmers and researchers alike could be that even though the AR monitoring techniques has been used for years, correlation between in vivo and in vitro tests for detecting BZ resistance is not always good [75]. This is probably because in vitro tests are more sensitive than in vivo tests [20], and those shortcomings concerning sensitivity and specificity could be subjugated by the use of molecular techniques than are not reliant on microscopy. In order to win the battle against the emergence of AR, correct use of anthelmintics and on-farm training about gastrointestinal helminths infecting livestock must be provided. Such training should be ongoing and provided by extension officers together with animal health technicians. Training initiatives should incorporate practical demonstrations and focus on aspects such as the importance of correct dosage, when to alternate anthelmintic classes and treatment frequency. Furthermore, a sustainable integrated parasite management must become the new paradigm, where anthelmintics are used much less frequently and in a more targeted and strategic manner following the principles of smart drenching and FAMACHA© together with a variety of nondrug-based practices. These strategies can be employed in combination with faecal egg counts.

Acknowledgements

The first author is supported by a grant holder bursary of the Collaborative Postgraduate Training Grant of the National Research Foundation (NRF) of South Africa (GUN: 105271) made available to OMMT.

Conflict of interests

The authors declare that they have no financial or personal relationships that may have inappropriately influenced them in writing this book chapter.

Declarations

The authors declare that all the literature and sources used in the writing of this book chapter have been properly cited in the text and in the reference section.

Author details

Morutse Mphahlele[1], Nthatisi Molefe[1], Ana Tsotetsi-Khambule[2] and Thekisoe Oriel[1*]

1 Unit for Environmental Sciences and Management, North-West University, Potchefstroom, South Africa

2 Department of Life and Consumer Sciences, College of Agriculture and Environmental Sciences, University of South Africa, Florida, South Africa

*Address all correspondence to: oriel.thekisoe@nwu.ac.za

References

[1] Van Dijk J, Sargison ND, Kenyon F, Skuce PJ. Climate change and infectious disease: Helminthological challenges to farmed ruminants in temperate areas. Animal. 2010;**4**:377-392

[2] Waller PJ. Sustainable nematode parasite control strategies for ruminant livestock by grazing management and biological control. Animal Feed Science and Technology. 2006;**126**:277-289

[3] Charlier J, Van der Voort M, Kenyon F, Skuce PJ, Vercruysse J. Chasing helminths and their economic impact on farmed ruminants. Trends in Parasitology. 2014;**30**:361-367

[4] Sanchez VVV, Patiño AS, Segundo VJP, Sandoval JACS, Esquivel CVC, Sanchez TAC. Prevalence of gastro-intestinal parasites among captive primates in Panama. Journal of Animal and Veterinary Advances. 2009;**8**:2644-2649

[5] Roeber F, Jex AR, Gasser RB. Impact of gastrointestinal parasitic nematodes of sheep, and the role of advanced molecular tools for exploring epidemiology and drug resistance: An Australian perspective. Parasites & Vectors. 2013;**6**:153

[6] Grisi L, Leite CR, Martins JRS, Barros ATM, Andreotti R, Cançado PHD, et al. Reassessment of the potential economic impact of cattle parasites in Brazil. Brazilian Journal of Veterinary Parasitology. 2014;**23**(2):150-156. DOI: 10.1590/S1984-29612014042. PMid:25054492

[7] Traversa D, Von Samson-Himmelstjerna G. Anthelmintic resistance in sheep gastrointestinal strongyles in Europe. Small Ruminant Research. 2015;**135**:75-80

[8] Kohler P. The biochemical basis of anthelmintic action and resistance. International Journal for Parasitology. 2001;**31**:336-345

[9] Mansour TE. Chemotherapeutic Targets in Parasites: Contemporary Strategies. Cambridge: Cambridge University Press; 2002. pp. 156-188

[10] Sangster NC, Dobson RJ. Anthelmintic resistance. In: Lee DL, editor. The Biology of Nematodes. London: Taylor & Francis; 2002. pp. 531-567

[11] Vercruysse J, Claerebout E. Overview of anthelmintics. In: The Merck Veterinary Manual. 2014. Retrieved from: http://www.merckvetmanual.com/mvm/pharmacology/anthelmintics/overview_of_anthel mintics.html

[12] Kotze AC, Hunt PW, Skuce P, Von Samson Himmelstjerna G, Martin RJ, Sager H, et al. Recent advances in candidate-gene and whole-genome approaches to the discovery of anthelmintic resistance markers and the description of drug/receptor interactions. International Journal for Parasitology: Drugs and Drug Resistance. 2014;**4**:164-184

[13] Oliveira-Sequeira TCG, Amarante AFT. Parasitologia animal: Animais de produção. 1st ed. Rio de Janeiro: EPUB; 2001

[14] Monteiro SG. Parasitologia na medicina veterinária. 1st ed. São Paulo: ROCA; 2011

[15] Baloyi MA, Laing MD, Yobo KS. Use of mixed cultures of biocontrol agents to control sheep nematodes. Veterinary Parasitology. 2012;**184**:367-370

[16] Geary TG, Hosking BC, Skuce PJ, Von Samson-Himmelstjerna G, Maeder S, Holdsworth WP, et al. WAAVP

guideline on anthelmintic combination products targeting nematode infections of ruminants and horses. Veterinary Parasitology. 2012;**190**:306-316

[17] Prichard RK, Hall CA, Kelly JD, Martins ICA, Donald AD. The problem of anthelmintic resistance in nematodes. Australian Veterinary Journal. 1980;**56**(5):239-251. DOI: 10.1111/j.1751-0813.1980.tb15983.x. PMid:7002142

[18] Drudge JH, Szanto J, Wyant ZN, Elam G. Field studies on parasitic control in sheep: Comparison of thiabendazole, ruelene, and phenothiazine. American Journal of Veterinary Research. 1964;**25**:1512-1518

[19] Jackson R, Rhodes AP, Pomroy WE, Leathwick DM. Anthelmintic resistance and management of nematode parasites on beef cattle-rearing farms in the North Island of New Zealand. New Zealand Veterinary Journal. 2006;**54**:289-296

[20] Overend DJ, Phillips ML, Poultion AL, Foster C. Anthelmintic resistance in Australian sheep nematode populations. Australian Veterinary Journal. 1994;**71**:117-121

[21] Ahmed M. Gastrointestinal (nematode) infections in small ruminants: Epidemiology, anthelmintic efficacy and the effect of wattle tannins [MSc thesis]. University of KwaZulu-Natal: Pietermaritzburg, South Africa; 2010

[22] Leathwick DM, Pomroy WE, Heath AC. Anthelmintic resistance in New Zealand. New Zealand Veterinary Journal. 2001;**49**:227-235

[23] Schnyder M, Torgerson PR, Schönmann M, Kohler L, Hertzberg H. Multiple anthelmintic resistance in *Haemonchus contortus* isolated from South African Boer goats in Switzerland. Veterinary Parasitology. 2005;**128**:285-290

[24] Cringoli G, Veneziano V, Rinaldi L, Sauve C, Rubino R, Fedele V, et al. Resistance of trichostrongyles to benzimidazoles in Italy: A first report in a goat farm with multiple and repeated introductions. Parasitology Research. 2007;**101**:577-581

[25] Burke J. Management of Barber pole Worm in Sheep and Goats in the Southern U.S. Booneville AR. Dale Bumpers Small Farms Research Update, n. p. 2005

[26] Anon. The World Factbook. CIA Directorate of Intelligence. 2007. Available from: http://www.cia.gov/ciapublicatins/pubs.html (Accessed: March 2007)

[27] Kaminsky R, Ducray P, Jung M, Clover R, Rufener L, Bouvier J, et al. A new class of anthelmintics effective against drug-resistant nematodes. Nature. 2008;**452**(7184):176-180. DOI: 10.1038/nature06722

[28] Jackson F, Coop RL. The development of anthelmintic resistance in sheep nematodes. Parasitology. 2001;**120**:95-107. DOI: 10.1017/S0031182099005740

[29] Van Wyk JA. Occurrence and dissemination of anthelmintic resistance in South Africa, and management of resistant worm strains. In: Boray JC, Martin PJ, Roush RT (eds). Resistance of parasites to antiparasitic drugs. Round Table Conference held at the VIIth International Congress of Parasitology, Paris; August 1990; MSD Agvet, Division of Merck, Rahway: New Jersey; 1990. pp. 103-113

[30] Van Wyk JA, Stenson MO, Van der Merwe JS, Vorster RJ, Viljoen PG. Anthelmintic resistance in South Africa: Surveys indicate an extremely serious situation in sheep and goat farming. Onderstepoort Journal of Veterinary Research. 1999;**66**:273-284

[31] Bakunzi FR. Anthelmintic resistance of nematodes in communually grazed goats in a semi-arid area of South Africa. Journal of the South African Veterinary Association. 2003;**74**:82-83

[32] Tsotetsi AM, Njiro S, Katsande TC, Moyo G, Baloyi B, Mpofu J. Prevalence of gastrointestinal helminths and anthelmintic resistance on small-scale farms in Gauteng Province, South Africa. Tropical Animal Health and Production. 2013;**45**:751-761

[33] Mukaratirwa S, Charakupa R, Hove TA. Survey of anthelmintic resistance on ten sheep farms in Mashonaland East Province, Zimbabwe. Journal of the South African Veterinary Association. 1997;**68**(4):140-143

[34] Matika O, Van Wyk JB, Erasmus GJ, Baker RL. Genetic parameter estimates in Sabi sheep. Livestock Production Science. 2003;**79**:17-28

[35] Boersema JH, Pandey VS. Anthelmintic resistance of trichostrongylids in sheep in the Highveld of Zimbabwe. Veterinary Parasitology. 1997;**68**(4):383-388. DOI: 10.1016/S0304-4017(96)01089-8

[36] Gabriel S, Phiri IK, Dorny P, Vercruysse J. A survey on anthelmintic resistance in nematode parasites of sheep in Lusaka, Zambia. Onderstepoort Journal of Veterinary Research. 2001;**68**:271-274

[37] Mwamachi DM, Audho JO, Thorpe W, Baker RL. Evidence for multiple anthelmintic resistance in sheep and goats reared under the same management in coastal Kenya. Veterinary Parasitology. 1995;**60**:303-313

[38] Voigt K, Scheuerle M, Hamel D. Triple anthelmintic resistance in *Trichostrongylus* spp. in a German sheep flock. Small Ruminant Research. 2012;**106**:30-32

[39] Domke AVM, Chartier C, Gjerde B, Hoglund J, Leine N, Vatn S, et al. Prevalence of anthelmintic resistance in gastrointestinal nematodes of sheep and goats in Norway. Parasitology Research. 2012;**111**:185-193

[40] McMahon C, Edgar HW, Barley JP, Hanna REB, Brennan GP, Fairweather I. Control of *Nematidirus* spp. infection by sheep flock owners in Northern Ireland. Irish Veterinary Journal. 2017;**70**:31. DOI: 10.1186/s13620-0109-6

[41] Artho R, Schnyder M, Kohler C, Torgerson PR, Hertzberg H. Avermectin resistance in gastrointestinal nematodes of Boer goat and Dorper sheep in Switzerland. Veterinary Parasitology. 2007;**144**:68-73

[42] Fortes FS, Kloster FS, Schafer AS, Bier D, Buzatti A, Yoshitani UY, et al. Evaluation of resistance in a selected field strain of *Haemonchus contortus* to ivermectin and moxidectin using the larval migration on agar test. Pesquisa Veterinaria Brasileira. 2013;**33**:183-187

[43] Rialch A, Vatsya S, Kumar RR. Detection of benzimidazole resistance in gastrointestinal nematodes of sheep and goats of sub-Himalayan region of northern India using different tests. Veterinary Parasitology. 2013;**198**:312-318

[44] Swarnkar CP, Singh D. Role of quarantine in management of anthelmintic resistance in strongyle worms of sheep. Indian Journal of Small Ruminants. 2012;**18**(1):95-99

[45] Kaplan RM, Vidyashankar AN. An inconvenient truth: Global worming and anthelmintic resistance. Veterinary Parasitology. 2012;**186**:70-78

[46] Papadopoulos E, Gallidis E, Ptochos S. Anthelmintic resistance in sheep in Europe: A selected review. Veterinary Parasitology. 2012;**189**:85-88

[47] Torres-Acosta JFJ, Mendoza-De-Gives P, Aguillar-Caballero AJ, Cuellarordaz JA. Anthelmintic resistance in sheep farms: Update of the situation in the American continent. Veterinary Parasitology. 2012;**189**:89-96

[48] Sangster NC, Cowling A, Woodgate RG. Ten events that defined anthelmintic resistance research. Trends in Parasitology. 2018;**34**:553-563. DOI: 10.1016/j.pt.2018.05.001

[49] Morgan ER. Detail and the devil of on-farm parasite control under climate change. Animal Health Research Reviews. 2013;**14**:138-142

[50] Sutherland IA, Leathwick DM. Anthelmintic resistance in nematode parasites of cattle: A global issue? Trends in Parasitology. 2011;**27**:176-181

[51] Sargison ND. Keys to solving problems in small ruminants: Anthelmintic resistance as a threat to sustainable nematode control. Small Ruminant Research. 2016;**142**:11-15

[52] Vijayasarathi MK, Sreekumar C, Venkataramanan R, Raman M. Influence of sustained deworming pressure on the anthelmintic resistance status in strongyles of sheep under field conditions. Tropical Animal Health and Production. 2016;**48**:1455-1462

[53] Čerňanská D, Várady M, Čudeková P, Čorba J. Worm control practices on sheep farms in the Slovak Republic. Veterinary Parasitology. 2008;**154**:270-276. DOI: 10.1016/j.vetpar.2008.03.026

[54] De Villiers JF, Gcumisa ST, Gumede SA, Thusi SP, Dugmore TJ, Cole M, et al. Estimation of live body weight from the heart girth measurement in KwaZulu–Natal goats. Applied Animal Husbandry and Rural Development. 2009;**1**:1-8

[55] Calvete C, Uriarte J. Improving the detection of anthelmintic resistance: Evaluation of faecal egg count reduction test procedures suitable for farm routines. Veterinary Parasitology. 2013;**196**:438-452

[56] Coles GC, Bauer C, Borgsteede FHM, Geerts S, Klei TR, Taylor MA, et al. World Association for the Advancement of Veterinary Parasitology (WAAVP) methods for the detection of anthelmintic resistance in nematodes of veterinary importance. Veterinary Parasitology. 1992;**44**(1-2):35-44. DOI: 10.1016/0304-4017(92)90141-U

[57] Coles GC, Jackson F, Pomroy WE, Prichard RK, von Samson-Himmelstjerna G, Silvestre A, et al. The detection of anthelmintic resistance in nematodes of veterinary importance. Veterinary Parasitology. 2006;**136**:167-185

[58] Vatta AF, Lindberg ALE. Managing anthelmintic resistance in small ruminant livestock of resource-poor farmers in South Africa. Journal of the South African Veterinary Medical Association. 2006;**77**:2-8

[59] Coles GC. Sustainable use of anthelmintics in grazing animals. Veterinary Record. 2002;**151**:165-169

[60] Lyndal-Murphy M, Swain AJ, Pepper PM. Methods to determine resistance to anthelmintics when continuing larval development occurs. Veterinary Parasitology. 2014;**199**(3-4):191-200. DOI: 10.1016/j.vetpar.2013.11.002

[61] Le Jambre LF. Egg hatch as an *in vitro* assay of thiabendazole resistance in nematodes. Veterinary Parasitology. 1976;**2**:385-391

[62] Elard L, Cabaret J, Humbert JF. PCR diagnosis of benzimidazole-susceptibility or -resistance in natural populations of the small ruminant parasite, Teladorsagia

circumcincta. Veterinary Parasitology. 1999;**80**:231-237

[63] Hubert J, Kerbouf DA. Microlarval development essay for the detection of anthelmintic resistance in sheep nematode. Veterinary Record. 1992;**130**:442-446

[64] Cala AC, Chagas ACS, Oliveira MCS, Matos AP, Borges LMF, Sousa LAD, et al. *In vitro* anthelmintic effect of *Melia azedarach* L. and *Trichilia claussenii* C. against sheep gastrointestinal nematodes. Experimental Parasitology. 2012;**130**:98-102

[65] Garcia LS, Arrowood M, Kokoskin E, Paltridge GP, Pillai DR, Procop GW, et al. Laboratory diagnosis of parasites from the gastrointestinal tract. Clinical Microbiology Reviews. 2018;**31**: e00025-17. DOI: 10.1128/CMR.00025-17

[66] Raymond M, Callaghan A, Fort P, Pasteur N. Worldwide migration of amplified insecticide resistance genes in mosquitoes. Nature. 1991;**350**:151-153

[67] O'Brien TF. The global epidemic nature of antimicrobial resistance and the need to monitor and manage it locally. Clinical Infectious Diseases. 1997;**24**:2-8

[68] Kwa MS, Veenstra JG, Roos MH. Molecular characterization of β-tubulin genes present in benzimidazole-resistant populations of *Haemonchus contortus*. Molecular and Biochemical Parasitology. 1993b;**60**:133-144

[69] Blouin MS, Yowell CA, Courtney CH, Dame JB. Host movement and the genetic structure of populations of parasitic nematodes. Genetics. 1995;**141**:1007-1014

[70] van Wyk JA. Refugia e overlooked as perhaps the most potent factor concerning the development of anthelmintic resistance. Onderstepoort Journal of Veterinary Research. 2001;**68**:55-67

[71] van Wyk JA, Hoste H, Kaplan RM, Besier RB. Targeted selective treatment for worm management-how do we sell rational programs to farmers. Veterinary Parasitology. 2006;**139**:336-346

[72] O'Shaughnessy J, Earley B, Mee JF, Doherty ML, Crosson P, Barrett D, et al. Nematode control in suckler beef cattle over their first two grazing seasons using a targeted selective treatment approach. Irish Veterinary Journal. 2015a;**68**:13

[73] Molefe NI, Tsotetsi AM, Ashafa AOT, Thekisoe OMM. *In vitro* anthelmintic activity of *Artemisia afra* and *Mentha longifolia* against parasitic gastro-intestinal nematodes of livestock. Bangladesh Journal of Pharmacology. 2012;**7**:157-163

[74] Waller PJ. International approaches to the concept of integrated control of nematode parasites of livestock. International Journal for Parasitology. 1999;**29**(1):155-164. DOI: 10.1016/S0020-7519(98)00178-7

[75] Dolinka M, Ivanisinova O, Königová A, Várady M. Anthelmintic resistance in sheep gastrointestinal nematodes in Slovakia detected by in-vitro methods. BMC Veterinary Research. 2014;**10**:233